SAY GOOD-BYE

TO

CHILDREN'S ALLERGIES

DATE DUE

SEP 1 0 2003		
OCT 0 2 2003		
NOV 2 4 2003		
DEC 1 7 2003		
JAN 0 6 2005		
APR 2 1 2006		
reviewed for c&c 10109 KEEP		
MAR 2 6 2011		
APR 1 9 2016		
AUG 2 3 2016		
GAYLORD		PRINTED IN U.S.A.

Web site: www.naet.com

DEDICATION

**This book is dedicated to all the parents
who are looking desperately for ways
to provide their children a healthier life**

First Edition: January, 2001

Copyright © 2001
by
Devi S. Nambudripad
D.C., L.Ac., R.N., Ph.D. (Acu)
Buena Park, CA

Library of Congress: 00-111258
ISBN: 0-9658242-8-4

Printed in U.S.A.

The medical information and procedures contained in this book are
not intended as a substitute for consulting your physician. Any attempt to
diagnose and treat an illness using the information in this book should
come under the direction of an NAET physician who is familiar with this
technique. Because there is always some risk involved in any medical
treatment or procedure, the publisher and author are not responsible for
any adverse effects or consequences resulting from the use of any of the
suggestions or procedures in this book. Please do not use this book if you
are unwilling to assume the risks. All matters regarding your health should
be supervised by a medical professional.

CONTENTS

NAET TESTIMONIALS

J.S. was a four year old boy who had suffered from a total body rash his entire life. He was very ill as an infant and in fact suffered from extreme allergies from the first day of life. At approximately two weeks of age he lost all of his skin in a massive shedding whereupon he was transferred to a university center where he battled for his life for several weeks.

When I first met the boy he had thick scales all over his body, many of which were red and angry looking. His mother was keeping him away from milk and eggs at that time as he had been R.A.S.T. tested. His problems at presentation were his marked eczema with scratching and sores which kept him from sleeping well, inability to go outside because of urticaria and chronic abdominal pains and diarrhea. He was so allergic to egg that even holding an unbroken egg would cause him to break out in hives (this was described as happening many times so I take it at face value).

He underwent NAET treatments going through the major foods and finally chemicals, pesticides and pollens. An interesting feature of his case is that he had IgE levels quantified before treatment and afterwards.

Allergens	Pre-treatment	Post treatment
Egg white	iv	1
Milk	iv	0

Allergens	Pre-treatment	Post treatment
Casein	iv	0
Total IgE	32	9.2

Today J.S. is a very happy boy. He can play outside anytime, eat what he wants and sleeps through the night without itching or special creams.

David M. Schultz, M.D.
Leipsic, OH (419) 943-2130

NAET works like a magic in some children. Often it can convert an irritable child from crying to smiling in minutes!

Mala Moosad, R.N., L.Ac.
Buena Park, CA (714) 523-8900

NAET is the most remarkable therapy I have ever experienced both professionally and personally. The transformation in those who suffer from debilitating chronic ailments, whether a young child or a senior, never cease to amaze me! And who would ever have suspected that the cause of their maladies were allergies? It is an honor to be doing this work - guiding people from a life of suffering to vitality! I thank Dr. Devi every day for creating such an amazing system of healing!.

Judit Rajhathy., B.A., R.N.C.P., D.Ac.
N.S., Canada (902) 466-0557

I enjoy treating Children with NAET. No needles or strange elimination diets. They love it!

Judith Abrams, L.Ac. PA-C
Ithaca, NY (607) 277-7713

At the age of three my son was classified as having PDD/Autism. After the shock wore off I decided to stop fighting with the pediatrician, and started listening to my family and friends to go the alternative way. When I learned about NAET I cried I was so happy. Needless to say I did what I had to, to get trained so I could treat my children. My children now 8 and 6 are no longer labeled autistic and attend regular schools. NAET is the answer to so many parents' prayers. Your child doesn't have to live a casein, gluten, food and chemical free life! I can't thank Dr. Devi Nambudripad and NAET enough for giving us our children back. Since two years I have started treating my autistic patients with NAET. I use NAET exclusively in my practice. Majority of my patients are children. I am so amazed in a short period of time how NAET has transformed many children's lives in my practice.

Maribeth Mydlowski, D.C.
Hamilton Township, NJ (609) 581-8484

Delayed growth and development, eczema, asthma, adverse vaccination reactions, behavior problems and sibling rivalry, ADD/ADHD and autism, diabetes, and digestive disorders, learning disability, ear infections, are just a few of the many pediatric conditions I have witnessed healed by NAET. This is truly a miraculous therapy.

Sandra Denton, M.D.
Anchorage, AK (907) 563-6200

NAET has given a new meaning to my practice when I treat young children. Practice has become more satisfying to watch the changes of my ADD children from being very hyperactive, impossible to calm, quiet, well balanced, lovable children.

Ann Mc Combs, D.O.
Seattle, WA (425) 576-0951

NAET has transformed the treatment of Pediatric illnesses in many of my cases. It's a great reward to hear a parent say: "I don't really understand this, but my daughter is turning into a neat young lady, and can eat many things she could not eat before!"

I thank you, "Dr. Devi," for bringing this remarkable addition into the armamentarium of the healing arts.

Peter R. Holyk, M.D., F.A.C.S.,
Sebastian, FL (561) 388-5554

NAET treatments in children in my practice have been a blessing to many of my patients and has been rewarding to me. It has specifically been used to remove lactose allergies causing colic symptoms in days and weeks old infants. NAET is also used successfully in removing allergies causing severe infantile eczema which otherwise would have to be treated with steroids. Additionally, the tremendous benefit is seen in the treatment of autism. By removing allergies these children are able to function better and it is certainly a blessing to these children and their families.

James Christianson, D.O.
Coffeyville, KS (419) 893-8438.

NAET has given me a fantastic technique in order to help my young patients. They look forward to coming into my office to get the tickling treatment.

Ranan Shahar, L.Ac.
Malibu, CA (310) 456-7721

"Kevin was unable to eat eggs. When he ate any products with eggs in them, his mouth turned into fire, his throat swelled, and he had to be rushed to the hospital ER or given an epipen injection. He was unable to enjoy birthday cakes and other delights made with eggs for four of his seven years. After his first NAET clearing for eggs, he was able to have a small portion of egg product. After clearing many combinations associated with eggs, including mayonnaise, cake frosting, stomach acid, grains and finally soybean oil and lecithin, Kevin is now able to eat any egg product — as much as he wants — without any reaction whatsoever. He's one very happy child, thanks to NAET!"

Dr. Gary Erkfritz, D.C.
Thousand Oaks, CA (805) 371-8082

Devi Nambudripad has pioneered the greatest leap in the field of energy medicine technology on the doorstep to the 21st Century, at a time when there is greater suffering from allergies than ever before. This book offers a glimpse into the miracles that NAET can bring to the lives of not only human children but of all creatures on the planet.

Roger Valentine, D.V.M.
Rahmie Valentine, L.Ac., O.M.D.
Santa Monica, CA (323) 936-3162

NAET is the most exciting thing happened to me in my 30 years of practice. I didn't believe allergies could be eliminated, but now thanks to Dr. Nambudripad's allergy elimination technique. I am able to change people's lives for the better by actually eliminating their allergies forever. Children no longer need to be "doped" or "drugged" through their youth.

David Pinkston, D.C.
Bishop, CA (760) 873-7178

Through NAET my patients have experienced extraordinary results in the elimination of their allergies.

Don Weiss, D.C.
Philadelphia, PA (215) 728-1413

Words cannot describe how valuable NAET is in working with children. The treatment is totally nonthreatening and painless. Children respond very quickly to NAET without experiencing unnecessary trauma. I am very grateful to Dr. Devi's commitment to this method of eliminating allergies.

Kathryn Ferrante,LTH.
Palm City, Fl (407) 297-0772

NAET is awesome... The traditional medical community needs to wake up and experience it's power.

Kerry Mac Rae, D.C.
San Francisco, CA (415) 567-2461

I have found NAET to work exceptionally well in children with inhalant and food allergies. They have been able to get along with the use of minimal medication. I have also seen remarkable improvement in children with asthma. There is a marked reduction in medication needed and most are able to take part in all regular activities.

Gerald D. Keyte, D.O., P.C.
Washington, MI (810) 781-5535

NAET has opened a new door to my young patients. My young ones are thrilled to have NAET, because they know that after one day's avoidance they can eat their favorite food.

Que Areste, N.D.
Seattle, WA (206) 328-2926

First I used NAET to treat the allergies of my child and my family. Now I have been using it on my patients, and virtually all of them have experienced significant improvement. NAET is the most important discovery of this century in the health field.

Eric Roth, M.D.
New York., NY (212) 253-0017

I have been practicing NAET for 10 years. It has changed my practice greatly and has affected many children's lives positively including many autistic children. Thank you Dr. Devi for helping me to make a difference in their lives.

Farangis Tavily, L.Ac
Mill Valley, CA (415) 302-7907

After retiring from psychiatry after practicing for over forty years, I must say that I have been pleasantly surprised at the dramatic results, which have occurred in my practice of the past few years. This has been especially true with pediatric patients.

A young girl was not able to play outdoors without developing severe eczema, but after NAET treatments for radiation was able to play outdoors with no problems. A twenty-month old girl had never stood or walked on her own, but she had successful surgery on both feet at age six months. After receiving NAET treatment for anesthesia, she stood alone for the first time several hours later, and was walking alone two days later. A six-week old boy had a rash on his face and was very irritable every time he nursed. He received NAET treatment for his mother's breast milk, then was more content immediately after he resumed nursing and his rash disappeared within a few days. A couple of teenage boys had been plagued with multiple asthmatic episodes, but, after each received a series of NAET treatments, they have now gone many months with no serious episodes.

These types of dramatic results, along with elimination of specific food allergies, make NAET stand out, in my opinion, as more effective than any other treatment program that has been developed up to this time in the history of mankind.

Robert M. Prince, MD.
NAET of North Carolina
Charlotte, NC (704) 844-8473

I have found NAET to be a very fast and effective tool in treating young children with allergies and hypersensitivities to foods, chemicals, environmental pollutants. I enjoy working with NAET.

Joe Seckel, M.A., H.P.
Sacramento, CA (916) 424-0242

NAET is a breakthrough and best treatment for allergies, pediatric problems and chronic ailments. Hundreds of our patients have regained their health through NAET.

Peter Gao, DAc., C.M.D., M.Sc.
Toronto, Ontario (416) 932-2802

I highly recommend Dr. Devi Nambudripad's Allergy elimination treatment for children. NAET provides me the best tool to uncover the difficult every day medical problem in children.

James Winer, D.C.
Pittsburgh, PA (412) 431-7246

After treating variety of health ailments in children with outstanding success, I can confidently say that NAET is the link we were missing in children's health care.

Debbie Carroll, R.N., L.Ac.
NB., Canada (506) 386-4866

NAET is a highly effective treatment for eliminating allergies in children. After the treatment, children are free to eat their favorite food without any adverse reaction. No needles, no pain!

Jacqueline Baschleben, D.C.
Roscoe, IL (815) 623-7694

I have used NAET successfully on my young patients. I have found NAET to be safe, effective, painless and very fast acting. I highly recommend its use to anyone who suspects that they must have allergies and/or food sensitivities.

Robert Ward, D.C.
Pocatello, ID (208) 232-2225

NAET is a life saving technique that is a must for all children. I treat children from new born to adolescents with excellent result. It is the best treatment for all types of allergies and allergy-related problems like skin conditions and behavioral problems. It is a very gentle technique, children love it.

David Hetzel, D.C.
Las Vegas, NV (702) 260-1164

Based on my experience and the results of thousands of NAET treatments in my clinic, I would like to state my observation that Dr. Nambudripad has elevated integrative medicine to a whole new level.

Gary Trott, L.Ac., O.M.D.
Bedford, TX (817) 285-0622

My hope is that parents come to realize that while most childhood illnesses such as ear infections, asthma, ADD, ADHD, are common, they are not conditions that children and their families need to cope with and accept. The first step to restoring a child's health is to reject the idea that these types of illnesses are normal. The second step is to let a child experience the self-healing that NAET induces.

Jacqueline Smillie, N.D.
Redlands, CA (909) 335-1980

NAET is amazing! One of my young patients was singing in a chorus. The house where she was practicing had a cat and she had to stand outside the house to practice since she was highly allergic to animals. She suffered from sneezing, hay-fever like symptoms and asthma when ever she came close to animal epithelial or dander. After she was treated and cleared for animal dander, epithelial and cat hair, she is very happy to join the choral group inside the house without any trace of her previous reactions.

Yvonne Tyson, M.D.
Long Beach, CA (562) 423-0436.

I love working with children. NAET has made my pediatric practice more pleasant. It is a fascinating technique of correcting children's allergies, which is an underlying cause of most pediatric health problems.

Marilyn Chernoff, N.D.
Albuquerque, NM (505) 292-2222

It is a joy to work with children using NAET. They respond well. Parents are impressed when they see improvement not only in their children's physical health but often in their behavioral problems as well.

Sue Anderson, D.C.,
Ann Arbor, MI (734) 662-9140

NAET is a major boom in the treatment of children with compromised immune system. I have also witnessed children with ADD and Autism make great progress.

Stefanie Pukit, D.C., C.C.H.
New York., NY (212) 206-8100

A four year old girl had bad stomach aches after ingesting milk, but after NAET treatments for basic allergens plus milk mix she told her mother "My stomach doesn't hurt now."

Salena Web. EMT. Psy. H.P.
NAET of North Carolina
Charlotte, NC (704) 844-8473

I have seen NAET transforming children with attention-deficit hyperactivity disorders into calm, responsible individuals. We have helped many children with ADD and ADHD in the past years with NAET.

Mohan Moosad, L.Ac
Buena Park, CA (714) 523-8900

NAET is a highly effective treatment for allergies and allergy-related health problems in children. I have received excellent results with my most difficult cases using NAET.

Mark Belnap, D.C.
Pocatello, ID (208) 232-2225

NAET has been an amazing tool to use on children with all sorts of otherwise hard to treat disorders. It is safe, effective, natural and painless. What a privilege to give children such a healthy head start in life!

Jan Viafora, D.C.
Sedona, AZ (520) 284-9550

I have seen a little girl who developed a bad rash on her buttocks every time she sat on her potty chair, who obtained immediate relief when her allergy to plastic was cleared. If it was not for NAET training, I wouldn't have been able to help her. NAET is amazing!

Iris Prince, R.N.
Charlotte, NC (704) 844-8473

I have treated hundreds of young patients with various ailments. I find great pleasure in watching how their lives change from a simple non-invasive technique.

Karen Berg,O.T., H.P.
Alexandria, VA (703) 354-7336

Using NAET, it's been possible to free people from the bondage of lifetime nutritional and environmental sensitivity. NAET has been a true blessing to so many.

Lawrence Bakur, D.C.
Green Village, NJ (914) 426-5588

I practiced Chinese Medicine for 20 years. However, after years of searching, I have found the missing link in testing allergies by integrating NAET into my practice for more complete and satisfactory outcome.

Iva Lim Peck, L.Ac. Dipl. Ac.,
Dallas, TX (972) 235-9070

NAET is the very effective treatment for food and environmental sensitivities. This is a quick, easy, non-invasive diagnostic test and the only treatment I have found that virtually eliminates food, chemical and environmental allergies. Since it is a painless, treatment, my pediatric patients love it.

Thomas Anderson, D.C.
Salt Lake City, UT (801) 272-9989

My young allergic clients respond quickly to NAET. Within hours of these individual treatments, appetite returns, emotions stabilize, and behavior patterns change drastically for the better. A parent's dream comes true through NAET!

Arianne Koven, N.D.
Palm Springs, CA (760) 328-1070

NAET is truly amazing! It allows me to give my patients freedom from pain and suffering that until now was not possible just by using the knowledge I learned in medical school alone. Not only that it bothered me to watch my patients return too frequently seeking care for the same problem. Now I realize that I was giving just temporary help to them. Since I added NAET to my practice, my patients are happier and I am too. Now I feel that I am doing something for my patients that is going to help them to live as productive individuals. Daily my patients tell me about their success stories they received from my NAET treatments that would be considered by most as "Miracles." NAET is not a "Miracle." It is hard work - hard work that gives you RESULTS! I wish all medical practitioners will learn NAET so that they all can provide their patients best of care by incorporating NAET into their existing practices without altering their present practices and derive utmost satisfaction from the results they see from their work. And for the patients? They too can have a normal life... they deserve it. Now it is possible through NAET. NAET is a must for all patients that suffer from allergies and allergy-related diseases. Thank you Dr. Devi for discovering NAET.

Jim Savor, D.C.
Allergy Relief Center, Herndon, VA

With pediatrics being a significant part of my practice, and having two daughters, Aryanna 7, and Shivani 3, I have not found anything under the sun in my 17 years of practice comparable to NAET. It's a miracle!

Roc H. Gantt, O.M.D., L.Ac., Dipl.Ac.
Sacramento, CA (916) 349-9223

I have treated patients from age two months to 70 years old and enormous pleasure in watching how their lives change from such simple acupuncture technique. One says, "I felt as if I was let out of Jail!" Another describes it as, "escape from allergy hell." My patients' improvement in health, mood and behavior are, in some cases, incredibly profound and the credit goes to NAET. Thank you Devi, for a technique that so quickly transforms so many lives.

Carolyn Reuben, L.Ac.
Sacramento, CA (916) 452-5887

Practicing NAET for the past 7 years has greatly enhanced both my professional and personal life. I have witnessed dramatic elimination of life threatening allergies, the routine reversal of bothersome allergies, and the gradual rebuilding of vitality and wellness from debilitating allergies in my young patients.

Andrew Pallos, DDS, L.Ac.
Laguna Niguel, CA (714) 495-6484

From my experience with several autistic children with whom I have recently worked, I have found that NAET provides a powerful tool to unravel the mystery of autism and restore a higher level of functioning. It gives hope where there was none before!

Susan LeFavour, LMSW, Ph.D.
Atlanta, GA (770) 643-6784

Terri, C.J.'s mother had come to me complaining of multiple food and environmental allergies. While I was treating her, she was getting great results, so she asked me about the possibility of treating her son for his asthma, behavioral problems and, especially, his anaphylactic reaction to peanuts. I told her I thought I could help him a great deal, so she brought him in and we started treating him also with NAET. I started by clearing him for all the basics, and then we did some environmentals that she knew were problems for him such as mold, dust, trees, weeds, grass, smoke, ragweed, flowers, perfumes, etc. At that point, I cleared him of some of the common foods that he ate such as tomatoes, potatoes, and spices. Then the time had come to clear for nuts, and, I have to be honest, I was a little apprehensive. He had been in the hospital several times with anaphylactic reactions to peanuts and I didn't want anything to happen to him. He cleared several times for both nut mixes and after we were sure he muscle tested strong for them, he ate peanut butter with no reaction!! At this point, not only was his allergy for peanuts gone, but also his asthma had improved dramatically and he was a very happy, well behaved child who has truly been a joy to be around. It is cases like this that make me eternally grateful to Dr. Devi Nambudripad for sharing her technique with me and hundreds of other practioners. Every day we make miraculous changes in the quality of people's lives. I can't imagine having a more rewarding career. Thank you, Dr. Devi!

Pamela Olson. D.C.
Elgin, IL (847) 888-0411

Dr. Devi's breakthrough approach of treating children's allergies is the perfect example of how alternative medicine can offer the perfect solution for allergy-related disorders. NAET helps you to identify the causes and allows you to not only eliminate them but also to lead a productive life.

Alan Bain, D.O.
Chicago, IL (312) 236-7010

NAET has provided me with a fast, effective allergy elimination technique to use with autistic children and those with severe development delays. This eliminates the need for extremely expensive blood profiles, rotation diets and desensitization shots. It is very beneficial in reprogramming brain frequency and lessening seizures. Dr. Devi is one of the few practitioners who understands the electromagnetic frequency of the body. As the paradigm of what the body "is" changes - so will the treatment modality. She is far ahead of her time. This is truly the MEDICINE OF THE FUTURE!

Pat Omiecinski, M.A., N.D., CNHP
Specialist for Autistic Children
Orlando, FL (407) 812-9446

At a time when food sensitivities, asthma, and environmental allergies in children are increasing at an alarming rate, NAET offers a safe, effective alternative to drug treatment that yields exceptional and lasting results.

Robert Sampson, MD, FAACAP
Andover, MA (978) 474-9009

Dr. Nambudripad's allergy elimination technique utilizes the unique autonomic nervous system regulating ability of acupuncture to desensitize the factors that are often the deep underlying causes of chronic illnesses. Children's nervous systems are particularly responsive to NAET often achieving good results in the treatment of most difficult conditions like asthma, attention-deficit hyperactive disorders, etc.

Richard Kitaeff, M.A., N.M.D., O.M.D.
Edmonds, WA 98020 (425) 775-6001

My first experience with allergy elimination was with Dr. Devi's Allergy elimination technique. It has changed the way I would practice for ever. When NAET is done properly it is very effective for allergy elimination. Our office incorporated NAET with our existing practice. NAET enhanced all my other practices and proved to be very very effective. After practicing for 31 years NAET has changed my practice and life for the better. I look forward to going to my office every day. Practice is more fun now since I incorporated NAET. You are never too old to learn or change what you are doing to be the most effective Doctor.

Michael E. Martin, D.C. N.M.D.
Topeka, Kansas (785) 228-1199

NAET is a highly effective treatment for allergies and allery-related health problems. I've received excellent results with my most difficult young patients using NAET

Jan Baumkel, D.O.
Ann Arbor, MI

NAET routinely provides safe, predictable, and durable responses in children of all ages. My own successful NAET cases range from a three month old premie with intolerance to all formula feedings to a 16 yr. old with anaphylactic reaction to peanuts, young asthmatics now free from their puffers, childhood allergic skin conditions, young children no longer subject to repeated ear infections, and ADD/ ADHD diagnosed students with improved grades and behavior. This is powerful work of interest to everyone who cares about improving the health of our children, and the efficacy of our healthcare system.

Leslie S. Feinberg, D.C.
Hermiston, OR (541) 567-0200

NAET is very effective for children and even infants, whether performed on the child or through a surrogate. Not only does the technique relieve and remove the child's allergies, but it reduces the burden on the parent for having to closely monitor their child's exposures. In children with untreated allergies, having other people give the child a food to which he/she is allergic is a parent's nightmare. In addition, treatment for chemicals makes it less mandatory to control the child's exposures to chemicals of all types.

Frances A. Taylor, M.A.
Los Alamos, NM 87544 (505) 662-9620

I highly recommend Say Good-bye to Children's Allergies to all parents. This book provides valuable guidance to help with your child's health problems.
Bess Liganor, M.D.
Internal Medicine, Pediatrics, Oncologist, Fresno, CA

ACKNOWLEDGMENTS

I am deeply grateful to my husband, Dr. Kris K. Nambudripad, for his inspiration, encouragement and assistance in my schooling and later, in the formulation of this project. Without his cooperation in researching reference work, revision of manuscripts, word processing and proofreading, it is doubtful whether this book would ever have been completed. My sincere thanks also go to the many clients who have entrusted their care to me, for without them I would have had no case studies, no technique and certainly no extensive source of personal research upon which to base this book.

I am also deeply grateful to the parents of my young patients Dominic, Steve, John, Steven, James, Matt, Brown, Mark, Ralph, Ann, Bob, Patrick, Eric, Paul, Young, John, Sean, Maureen, peyton, Margaret, and Nitya and all other children whose names I haven't mention here due to lack of space, for believing in me from the very beginning of my research, supporting my theory and helping me conduct the on-going *detective* work.

I also like to thank Prasad, Sara, Nathan, Karthik, Peyton and their parents for allowing me to take pictures to share with others for educating them about NAET.

I like to express my heartfelt thanks to my friends who are excellent NAET practitioners who supported me by providing case studies, patients' testimonials, and constant encouragements to bring this book out. Without their ardent help, the writing of this book would have remained just a dream.

Additionally, I wish to thank Mala, and Mohan for allowing me to work on the book by relieving me from the clinic duties, and helping me in the formulation of this book I do not have enough words to express my thanks to Chi Yu Tien, Fong Tien, and many of my friends who wish to remain anonymous for proofreading the work, and Mr. Sridharan at Delta Publishing for his printing expertise.

I am deeply grateful for my professional training and the knowledge and skills acquired in classes and seminars on chiropractic and applied kinesiology at the Los Angeles College of Chiropractic in Whittier, California; the California Acupuncture College in Los Angeles; SAMRA University of Oriental Medicine, Los Angeles; all my teachers at these universities and the clinical experience obtained at the clinics attached to these colleges.

I extend my sincere thanks to these great teachers. They have helped me to grow immensely at all levels. My mentors are also indirectly responsible for the improvement of my personal health as well as that of my family, patients and other NAET practitioners among whom are countless doctors of western and oriental medicine, chiropractic, osteopathy, as well as their patients.

Many of the nutritionists instrumental in this process, were professors at the institutions I have mentioned. Their willingness to give of themselves to teach, as well as their commitment of personal time to give the interviews necessary to complete this work, places them beyond my mere expressions of gratitude. They are servants to the greatest ideals of the medical profession.

Dr. Devi S. Nambudripad
Los Angeles, CA

FOREWORD

BY

David I Minkoff, M.D.

Clearwater, Florida

This book presents about commonly
seen pediatric allergies and how you can help your child to
get rid off them and thus help your child grow up healthy
and happy using natural means of health resorces such as
acupuncture, acupressure,
chiropractic,
nutrition, and herbs

FOREWORD
by
David I. Minkoff, M.D.

In 1974, I started a rotating internship in San Diego, California. While doing my first rotation in the Pediatric department, Dr. Allen, the director of the program, came up to me one day and said he wanted to have a meeting with me. When I got into his office he said, "What area of medicine are you going to go into?"

"I'm not really sure," I said. "I can't decide. That's why I thought if I did the rotating internship and learned a little about each subject I would know better, by the end of the year, what I wanted to do." Without hesitation, he looked up at me and said "You'd make a good pediatrician. Why not do that?" "Really?" I said. "You bet," he said. I said "Okay, I will!" And I did. Pediatrics was fun. It was the kids. It was that they usually got better. I had a ball.

One of the most fun things to do as a pediatrician is to help a child get well. Once you've done that with a family, they know you can do it again and again. Their trust in you is the real joy of practice. You can solve problems. You can get people well--usually.

Yet sometimes, this goal was elusive. Another ear infection, another cold, another sleepless night, another diarrheal stool. "Gosh Mrs. Jones, this is Katie's 5th ear infection this year and her 5th round of antibiotics." Then my certainty would become hesitant. "Is this right?" I would think. But I would be reassured by my journals that said by the time an average U.S. child is 5 years old they would have been on antibiotics 45 times!

I would scratch my head and think, well we just have to do it. She has a high fever, is ill, can't chance it going to her brain or blood, so we have to do it. I am a specialist in Pediatric Infectious disease. This is how we do it. No one would question this logic. But it gnawed on me when I would look at the chart: Amoxil, then Septra, then Zithromax, then Ceclor, and then Augmentin. Wow, a lot of medication. Can this be good? Then tubes in the ears, then the tonsils and adenoids out, then allergy shots. And with the same blind logic then Ritalin, and Cylert, Tegretal and Dilantin and ...and........

For the vast majority of MD's in this country the logic is never questioned. It is how it is done, standard of care and all that. That was my standard for my first 23 years of practice. "It is how we do it."

Then I met Devi Nambudripad and my medical life, my logic, and my practice got an awakening. You mean an infection could be caused by a blocked energy flow in the body? A blocked energy flow could be caused by chi not flowing? This was a sympathetic-parasympathetic imbalance, which was caused by an outside substance that created this response in the body, when it is near the body or eaten? This is truly what allergy is? And this leads to mucous, which leads to blocked up ducts, and blocked up ducts lead to ear infections? Oh my God.

Does NAET work? Can it end the cycle of drug after drug after drug for: runny nose, ear infections, poor bowel habits, menstrual cramps, behavior problems and hyperactivity? The answer is yes. NAET is the pediatricians best weapon. It is the medicine of the future----now. Ampicillin step aside. Ritalin -- dimetapp--wait a while-- I use drugs sparingly in my practice now. Before I prescribe any drug, vitamins or other supplements, I use NAET to test the compatibily, any possible adverse reaction, dosage and number of days required to get the maximum benefit. You will be surprised to see how the allergy-free drugs/supplements work like magic.

The body is a coherent system. This means it has logic, will regulate itself, and can heal itself if given the proper direction. NAET testing finds the blockage in the system. The treatment opens it allowing the system to fix itself. Drugs NEVER fix the system. They may temporarily help it, or cover up one's perception of it, or the symptom. But it doesn't fix it. NAET fixes it. Then it will run normally.

This is good medicine. And it is satisfying medicine. Because after an NAET treatment it looks like a miracle happened. I think all of us as doctors want to produce miracles. As an NAET M.D., I produce them on a daily basis. My patients have grown to expect it. "I can eat peanut butter now," stated a 6-year-old Jamie, "and that makes me happy." "That makes me happy too," I told him. As physicians we must be continually students. And as students we are lucky to meet a teacher whose vision of life is broader and more complete than ours. For in that relationship there are rich lessons to be learned.

For me, Devi is one of those teachers. Her message of health is carried by thousands of doctors to tens of thousands of patients every day. Modern pediatric practice can be dangerous for children. With NAET we have a safe science. I hope that every practitioner who cares for children will read her books, learn NAET, and use it to make the world a happier and healthy place.

David I. Minkoff M.D.
Diplomat American Board of Pediatrics
Fellow American Academy of Pediatrics
Subspecialty in Pediatric Infectious Disease
Lifeworks Wellness Center
Clearwater, Florida. (727) 466-6789

PREFACE

PREFACE

There is a myth among lay people all over: if a child didn't get sick while growing up, he/she would have poor immunity as an adult. Until recently everyone including many professionals believed in that myth to hold some truth. But no one realized the in-depth involvement of allergies in the increasing number of childhood diseases. In most cases allergies were inherited and in some they were acquired after the children were born. In any case, most children suffered from numerous allergies from birth and with the result, they suffered from multitudes of childhood illnesses in varying degrees and intensities soon after they were born.

If you could take time to run an investigation on the health history of various grown up people among us from different walks of life, you would be surprised to find how many lives are molded in how many different ways due to the unforseen impact of allergies of all kinds. It could make you sad and depressed for days when you realize the potential outcome of these people. They would all be leading different lives now if their allergies were corrected immediately as they were expressed or manifested in their mildest forms in their childhood. Can you imagine the effects of simple food and environmental allergies in young children leading to severe health problems in later lives? Some of these common childhood problems have been followed from childhood days to adulthood and the results have been very painful. If our health care system would look into educating all health care professionals everywhere about the influences of simple allergies in everyone's lives, if we train them to nip them in the bud, we would have a healthy population around us. Allergies appear and affect people in many ways; we need to look for them to find them. You may not find them until you realize that allergies may be causing frequent attacks of everyday common colds and flu's to severe asthma; mild itching and hives or skin rashes to severe eczema; poor concentration and mild learning disability to severe attention deficit disorders and autism; mild temper tantrums and mood swings to severe depression and suicide attempts; or unaddressed mild behavioral problems in childhood ending up in severe criminal activities as adults.

The study of allergies showed me the fascinating relationship between food and environmental allergies and many physiological and psychological problems. The limited research of allergies conducted so far has made this information available to a few who treat allergies and to the patients who have undergone the treatments. I like to show how the allergies affected various people in one of the families I treated since 1985 (soon after I began my allergy practice on patients) and the affects of NAET through four generations. The real names of the patients have been replaced with fictitious names to maintain privacy.

Karen and Sharon were sisters. Karen suffered from asthma ever since her childhood. She was fifty-one years old when she came to me for NAET. She suffered from at least one moderate to severe asthmatic attack everyday in spite of all her prescription medications she was taking daily for her breathing difficulties. As a child she suffered from frequent bronchitis and pneumonia and later she developed nasal polyps. She had multiple surgeries over the years to remove the polyps in the past since the polyps grew back to the original size every couple of years increasing the agony of breathing along with her lifetime companion - asthma.

Her family history revealed that her mother suffered from severe arthritis and father from severe asthma all his life until his death a few years ago.

She began NAET and by the time she was treated for basic ten, her asthma was under control. She was able to reduce the cortisone and other medications to a minimum dosage.

When Karen received such outstanding results with NAET in such a short time, she convinced her whole family to be my patients. She and her family thought NAET worked like magic. (They still think it does!).

Sharon suffered from severe migraines and frequent sciatic pains. She was also on various prescription medications for years. Her migraines were relieved by the time she was treated for sugar mix. Obviously her migraines were triggered by sugar allergy. But her sciatic pain continued without a change even after basic 15 treatments. According to her history, the pain usually began on her left hip around 8:00 to 9:00 am and radiated into her left thigh, knee, and ankle sometimes even to the fourth and fifth toes by evening. She worked between 9:00 to 5:00 P.M. in an office. Often it was hard to drive home in spite of all the pain medications she took and lumbosacral support she wore to control pain. Her puzzled doctors took various X-rays including scans but to their amazement everything turned out to be negative. Sharon was very intelligent and an efficient office manager of a big law firm. She was also evaluated for psychosomatic disorders and also treated by a special clinic for pain management, but none gave her any relief of her sciatic pain. Her doctors asked her to get disability, but her strong will power forced her to refuse that path. She made good money at her work. A single mother of two girls who owned three cars and a home in a plush neighborhood couldn't afford to be on disability. She decided to fight until she succeeded. She was also seeing a chiropractor regularly. Adjustments and ultrasound massages helped her temporarily for a couple of hours or so and helped her to sleep better on the days of the chiropractic treatments. She said that was the only thing which gave her some significant relief even if it only lasted for a couple of hours. She was so desperate to get relief from her pain and she was also treated by someone for past life traumas. But pain returned every morning with full intensity.

In our office we treated her for all the possible environmental allergens including grasses, pollen, weeds, dust, cotton, polyester, acrylic, animal dander and epithelial, etc. But in spite of all these treatments, she continued to have the same pain pattern - beginning in the morning and easing slightly by night.

I was very new with NAET. I was actually in the learning process. These were some of my pioneer patients who helped me to form NAET and give structure and shape to

NAET. I had no idea of the potentials of NAET. I didn't ask any questions. I moved towards the directions where I was led by the situations. I was a willing explorer. I firmly believe that all the opportunities for NAET opened to me by becoming just an open-minded willing explorer.

I was at my wit's end with Sharon when I decided to probe into her sciatic pain closely. I asked her to pinpoint the exact location of the origin of the pain on her body and she pinpointed to a specific point around left side of her hip over her denim pants. I slowly lowered her jeans on the side of the pain to take a close look at the location of the pain. Suddenly my eyes stared at the name tag of the pants rubbing against the skin of the side of the hip - the exact location of the origin of pain! I muscle tested her for the name tag. She was extremely allergic to it. I removed the tag carefully including the thread that was used on it and treated her immediately using NAET. She always wore jeans. She had no other clothes to wear. She was sent home in one of our fancy office gowns that evening after treatment.

On the third day she barged into my office with a big smile. She exclaimed, "We did it this time, Dr. Devi, Thank You!"

That was the end of her years-long sciatic pain. I didn't see her again for a long time.

This opened my eyes too. I began looking into every little object around the patient if the problems persisted. One becomes a detective when you work with NAET.

A couple of months later I got a phone call from Sharon. She was sobbing and muttering something that I couldn't clearly understand. All I could hear was that she needed an appointment right away and I said okay. I was so certain that her sciatic pains had returned.

It was just a few minutes after five in the evening when she showed up with her older daughter Sandy.

Sharon and Sandy both had swollen faces and reddish looking muddled eyes. One look at them and I knew there was something terribly wrong. I waited for them to speak up.

Sharon all of a sudden broke into crying spells and I put my arms around her. Sandy sat down in the chair crying too.

After a moment's pause, I asked, "Do you want to talk?"

"Our dreams all shattered, Dr. Devi," she said between her sobs. "We work so hard to live like normal people and when we think we are almost making it, everything crumbles down. We were so happy that finally we conquered my sciatic pain and now God gives us another blow. Sandy has been diagnosed as having multiple sclerosis by UCLA and we got the report yesterday."

Sandy was 22, married three months ago, and she was a beautician, worked all day, seven days a week.

Sandy burst into tears now. I handed her a tissue and sat next to her. I asked calmly, "Now tell me when did all this start?" I paused for a moment. Last time when I saw you, it was just before your wedding, you had no complaints, did you?"

I remembered Sandy accompanying Sharon one time into my office before her wedding. She appeared to be normal at that time.

"I had no complaints until two months ago," said Sandy. The first thing I noticed was weakness of both of my arms. Then I began having burning pains from neck down radiating into both arms. The pain was very mild in the beginning and it got progressively worse. I began dropping things frequently. Even the lightest things I couldn't hold without dropping. I was afraid to tell anyone about my problem. Tom was very observant. He noticed my struggle. He made an appointment with our internist. He referred me to UCLA. They ran a number of tests during the past week and finally it is confirmed now that I have MS."

I looked at her in disbelief with her diagnosis. I couldn't find any indication of MS in her energy channels. She had a huge angry looking pimple on her nose indicating the stomach and spleen meridians' dysfunction. Dark shadows on both sides of her cheeks indicated liver toxicity. Her chin was clear and had no dark circles under her eyes indicating no disturbance in the kidney meridians. Usually energy blockages are seen on kidney meridians when someone suffers from true multiple sclerosis.

I got up from my chair and told her, "Let me do some testing on you to see if you have true MS or allergies mimicking MS." I added, " If you have just allergies, then there is nothing to worry since we can treat them with NAET."

I saw Sharon closing her eyes for a moment; she was praying silently, then she said, "From your mouth to God's ears!"

I tested her using MRT and QRT (Question-response testing) for all the basic allergens. She was highly allergic to all of them. QRT also revealed that she was highly allergic to nuts and the nut allergy was causing the MS like symptoms.

"Do you eat a lot of nuts?" I enquired.

"None at all." She said.

"Are you sure about that?" I raised my eyebrows. "My kinesiological testing shows that you are eating lots of nuts daily for the last 10 weeks."

"I am eating lots of trail mix lately." She said. "In fact I think there are nuts in the trail mix and I am eating lots of those now-a-days."

"What is trail mix?" I asked. How much more ignorant can I be?

She opened her handbag and pulled out a zipped plastic bag with some food in it. I opened the bag to examine the contents. It had dried dates, raisins, almond flakes, split pea-nuts, sunflower seeds, and pieces of some other dried fruits.

"Sandy," I said confidently, "I think you are simply allergic to the nuts in this trail mix." I looked into her eyes confidently and said, "I don't think you have multiple sclerosis according to my testing."

She jumped out of the table to hug me. Then she hugged Sharon and they both cried for a few minutes.

I told her not to eat that trail mix again until she is treated satisfactorily. But she had to go through all the basics before I could treat her for the trail mix. Next few days she visited my office regularly. When she stopped eating the convenient health food, her symptoms of multiple sclerosis began to subside. After the basics I began treating her for nuts. All her previous symptoms returned. She also developed an extra complaint: burning sensation inside her brain.

She complained every time I treated her with nuts, "My brain is burning, I can't take it anymore." Certainly, her weak area of the body was brain. She complained of "brain burning" every time I gave her NAET. But she said her burning got better 25 hours after the treatments. But it returned after the next treatment. This pattern continued. Her MRT (muscle response testing) got strong soon after the treatment and continued to stay strong for a couple of hours but could not hold it for 25 hours. So the treatments for nuts had to be repeated at every visit and it took three months to pass the treatment for nut mix 1 and 2 - at the rate of three NAET treatments per week. *The more severe the allergies, the longer the treatments!*

Her symptoms were almost gone by the time she passed the nuts. But when we began vegetable and animal fats, her symptoms returned. It took another three months for her to pass all fats (vegetable fats, animal fats and fatty acids).

By then her liver spots on the face cleared up, spleen and stomach cleared up, her energy was normal. Her pains on the shoulders and arms went away. She didn't drop things any more. She returned to UCLA to have another check up. She got the report that her MS was in remission. Her doctors didn't have any explanation. She did not tell them anything about nut allergies and NAET, because I instructed her not to do so. They would not have believed her. Fifteen years later, we still face huge problems to make anyone understand NAET. How could we have explained anything to them then?

Fifteen years later, her MS remains still in remission.

Two years later, I had another phone call from Sharon and said she needed an appointment for Sandy. Sandy and Sharon came in next day. Sandy was seven months pregnant. But she had a rather disturbing news. Her body was making antibodies against the fetus. She was getting severe unbearable cramps in the abdomen. Her gynecologist was observing her for the past one month and she wasn't getting any better. Finally her doctor advised her to induce the labor and she told Sandy that her main obligation at that time was to save the mother. That was on a Thursday. Doctor suggested the induction procedure to be held as soon as possible since the antibody productions were rising fast and it could endanger the mother's life.

Sandy and Tom had dreamed great things for this baby. They prayed that something would happen to save their baby and alter the doctor's decision.

Sandy continued to get frequent severe cramps as we were discussing the pregnancy history. She was treated for all the NAET basics two years ago. I retested all her previous treatments and everything that was on the treated list tested fine. More NAET MRT and QRT were performed. She was found to be allergic to the fetus by MRT. More than that she was found to be allergic to her sweat suit she was wearing. The MRT showed that the allergy to the sweat pant was the cause of the abnormal antibody production.

"How long ago have you started wearing this outfit and how often do you wear this?" I questioned her.

"I bought this one about three months ago ." She added, "This is so comfortable and feels very soft against my growing tummy. So I bought three more pairs in different colors and I practically wear this kind all the time, even to bed at night."

They traveled two hours to see me. It was not possible to send her home to change clothes before I treated her. So I suggested to her to go to a nearby store and buy a set of non-allergic clothes before the treatment and she did so.

She was treated for her sweat suit, then later for the allergy to her fetus. Sandy returned on Saturday for retest and she was all smiles. She said she did not have any more cramps after the treatments for an allergy to the fetus and the sweat suit on Thursday.

She saw her gynecologist on Monday and reported that she had no more cramps and she told her about NAET treatments and the results. Her doctor was very happy and postponed the planned surgical procedure. A week later the blood test for the antibodies showed that she had no more antibody activities in her body against the fetus.

Sandy carried to full term without any more complications and gave birth to a healthy 8 lbs handsome boy. When she was pregnant with her second child, her gynecologist insisted to test for antibodies in her blood against the fetus, since it is quite common to expect something like that. But doctor was surprised at the normal report.

She stayed in the hospital for three days after the delivery. Then she and her son were sent home.

The new colorful nursery, a brand new baby crib, crib full of toys and ornaments greeted little Steven. Baby was nursed well and Sandy placed him in the crib to sleep. He was so beautiful and comfortable in the blue outfit. She kept looking at him with admiration and love for this little one. A few minutes into his sleep she was still looking at him and she couldn't take her eyes off of him. All of a sudden her keen eyes noticed something unusual. His pink lips were getting bluish. She looked at his chest and he wasn't breathing. She shook him and he wasn't waking up. She called 911 immediately and took the baby out of the crib into her arms. Tom, a paramedic himself, got to her side quickly and began CPR on him. By the time the emergency help arrived, they revived little Steven.

He was taken back to the hospital for observation. In the hospital he behaved okay. After 24 hours, he was sent home with a monitor and an alarm to alert any more such incidences.

Back in his own crib, he had another attack of sleep apnea just in a few minutes. Each time the alarm tripped, Sandy would shake him and wake him up. He had four more attacks repeatedly every few minutes. They had to call 911 again and take him back to the hospital. In the hospital he behaved normal but once at home, he acted the same.

They had to take him to the hospital emergency four times during his seven days in the world. On the seventh day Sandy realized he may be allergic to something in the house that was causing his sleep apnea. She brought little Steven to me straight from the hospital for evaluation. He was found to be allergic to all the plastic and formaldehyde products. He was allergic to the crib, the new baby mattress, pillow, plastic covering of the mattress, crib toys, ornaments, and other decorative objects on the crib. Sandy was never treated for plastic or formaldehyde before. Even though her mother was highly allergic to formaldehyde, since Sandy did not show any reaction towards it, that was left untreated. But little Steven expressed extreme allergy towards the formaldehyde. Amazingly, he was not allergic to the items Sandy was treated during pregnancy.

He was treated for all those items one by one. They bought non-allergic clothes and materials for the crib and removed all the toys and ornaments until they were sure that he was free of allergies to every little items. Little Steven and his loving parents were happy once again.

Little Steven is a 12 year-old healthy teenager now.
This is the story of one family I have treated since 15 years. I have treated many families with many such unique problems during my 17 years of NAET practice. This clearly shows allergies and allergic tendencies are inherited or handed down to younger generations by their ancestors.

I have given a number of commonly seen allergy-based pediatric problems and some immediate solutions for them in chapters 5 & 6 along with a few case studies. These are some of the common pediatric ailments you see in your daily life among our children. These are selected from my practice. I have treated variety of allergy-based childhood ailments with great results. Allergies are not considered real sickness. But people who suffered or are still suffering will know how miserable and devastating allergies can be. When my child was little he was sick almost every day with something or other. No doctor ever told me that he had allergies.

I went from one pediatrician to another, sat in their busy offices many hours at a time seeking some assistance in relieving his immediate problems like nasal congestion, fever, diarrhea, constipation, hives, rashes, vomiting, earaches, ear infection, abdominal pains, insomnia, leg pains, etc. etc. The list of my son's pediatric problems could go on. Now when I look back, I could say that he was a universal reactor. A few times I had to return home in tears without seeing the doctor because he had to run to the hospital delivery room, because another new child was arriving without previous warning and all the waiting room patients had to be rescheduled for another day. Years of struggle with my son's illnesses, desperation to find a cure for his problems, frustration of not finding any help from anywhere, finally led me to read and learn as much information as possible in medical fields (herbal, allopathic and natural home remedies). Finally God heard my prayers, understood my frustration and led me to NAET. While I was frantically searching for some help for my child's problems, I determined in my mind that if I ever found any help, I would make sure that I share the information with all other mothers of the world who are frantically, desperately, looking for some help with their darling children's health problems so that they all do not have to travel the same ugly road I had to long time ago.

The helpful home remedies I have given in this book are taken from my collection. I do not remember the sources where I got them from. I was not careful to write them down. I sincerely appologize for not giving appropriate credit for the sources. I wrote them down, tried them out and found them quite effective. You are free to use them and try them out yourself and see the results.If you are satisfied, please share with other mothers. That is my only request- from a mother to another mother!

Allergic manifestations may change from person to person depending on his/her particular weakness in the body. For example: if the brain is the weak area, allergies could affect the brain causing brain symptoms (anger, depression, ADD, ADHD, Autism, behavioral problems, personality disorders, etc.); If the lungs are the weak areas, allergies could affect the respiratory system causing respiratory disorders (SIDS, bronchitis, pneumonia, colds, flu's, cough, etc.), and so on. Please refer to Chapter 9 for the effect of allergies causing pathological symptoms of the weak meridians and organs.

As I began to realize how prevalent the problem of allergies was, and started to show effective results with my patients, I decided to write a book that would be informative to both health professionals and lay people. This book offers nearly the identical information as the dissertation for my doctorate degree, which compared oriental and western medical treatments for allergens. However, the text here is focused on describing the latest in allergy treatments in a way that can be understood by anyone interested in the topic. It is meant to help allergy sufferers understand more about their allergic reactions and know more about possible treatments. Technical terminology, although occasionally necessary, is kept to a minimum. I've also avoided getting into too much depth in areas that are extremely complex. Consequently, for example, I've stressed the important connection between the nervous system and allergic reactions without going into an in-depth analysis of the nervous system.

My real purpose in writing this book is to help my readers and through them their young ones achieve and maintain good health through treatments that are available to everyone today. In addition to this text, the companion books, Say Good-bye to Illness, The NAET Guide book, and Living Pain Free with Acupressure, (a book that shows the reader how to give themselves acupressure to reduce pain and get temporary help in various areas through acupressure) may also provide information that can help the reader to understand and alleviate his/her pain or discomforts. Additional information can be gathered by reading the books and articles referred to in this book's bibliography.

As chiropractic, acupuncture and Chinese herbs are the focal points of the treatments described in this and my other books, this book explains some of the basic tenets of energy blockages, nerve impingements and concise and simple explanation of acupuncture, Traditional Chinese Medicine (TCM), and herbs. However this book is not meant to give an in-depth understanding of chiropractic, or oriental medicine. Readers are encouraged to study more if they are interested to acquire more knowledge in these areas. Some references for more detailed reading of these subjects are also listed in the bibliography.

Stay allergy free and enjoy better HEALTH!

Dr. Devi S. Nambudripad,
D.C., L.Ac., R.N., Ph.D. (Acu.)
Los Angeles, California
January, 2001
(714) 523-8900

INTRODUCTION

Say Good-bye To Children's Allergies

YOUR CHILD DESERVES PERFECT HEALTH!

It is your child's human right to eat whatever he/she wants, live in whatever environment he/she wants to live, wear whatever clothes or cosmetics he/she wants to wear, live or associate with whomever he/she wants to and be happy. If your child is able to do all these things, your child is healthy physically, physiologically and psychologically, and if not, your child has an illness. This book will help you find your child's source of illness and assist you in finding the right help for your child in order to achieve perfect health.

This book reveals a remarkable breakthrough in medical history. It brings a breath of fresh air to the medical field and approaches health care from a new intelligent view.

This book is filled with common sense that it simply cannot be ignored by anyone who wants to be healthy. The central nervous system reacts to food or other substances around your child as if they are toxic when they are really neutral or beneficial for growth and development. You can now reprogram your brain to accept these good things of life as beneficial items to the body and achieve perfect health.

You'll learn how genetically passed energy blocks, which create adverse reactions, can now be removed -- doing away with the causes of most illnesses, perhaps all of them.

Kinesiology, chiropractic, acupressure and acupuncture

techniques have already been proven and accepted in the medical world. It is important to note that these procedures along with Dr. Nambudripad's discovery will be beneficial to all mankind.

What is NAET?

NAET is a short form for Nambudripad's Allergy Elimination Techniques. Various effective parts of healing techniques from different disciplines of medicine (allopathy, acupuncture, chiropractic, kinesiology and nutrition) have been compiled together to create NAET, to permanently eliminate allergies of all kinds (food and environmental allergies and reactions in varying degrees from mild to severe to anaphylaxis) from the body. NAET is a completely natural, non-invasive, drug-free holistic treatment. Over four thousand licensed medical practitioners have been trained in NAET procedures and are practicing all over the world. Please look up the NAET website for more information on NAET and a NAET practitioner near you. Our Website address is:

WWW.naet.com

What is an allergy?

A condition of unusual sensitivity of one individual to one or more substances (may be inhaled, swallowed, or came in contact with the skin), which may be harmless or even beneficial to the majority of other individuals. In sensitive individuals, contact with these substances can produce a variety of symptoms in varying degrees ranging from slight itching to swelling of the tissues and organs, mild runny nose to severe asthmatic attacks, general tiredness or fatigue to severe anaphylaxis. The ingested, inhaled or contacted allergen is capable of alerting the immune system of the body. The frightened and confused immune system then commands the white blood cells to produce immunoglobulins type E (IgE) to stimulate the release of the chemical defense forces like histamines from the mast cells. These chemical mediators are released as part of body's immune response to the foreign substances and these chemicals produce abnormal physical, physiological and psychological symptoms in the sensitive person.

What Causes Allergies?
1. Heredity
2. Toxins
3. Low Immune System
4. Radiation
5. Emotional factors

What Are Some Common Allergens?
Inhalants: pollens, flowers, perfumes, chemicals, dust, etc.
Ingestants: food, drinks, vitamins. drugs, additives, etc.
Contactants: fabrics, cosmetics, furniture, bed, toys, etc.
Injectants: insect bites, injectable drugs, vaccinations, etc.
Infectants: bacteria, virus, contact with infected persons.
Physical Agents: heat, cold, humidity, dryness, wind, etc.
Genetic Agents: inherited illnesses or tendency from parents, grand parents and ancestors.
Molds, Fungi: yeast, candida, molds, parasites, etc.
Emotional Factors: painful memories of various incidents from past or present.

How Do I know If my child has Allergies?

If your child experiences or demonstrates any unusual physical, physiological or psychological symptoms in the presence of any of the above items, you can suspect an allergy.

Who Should Use This Book?

Anyone with a child who is suffering from food, chemical and environmental allergies or allergy-related diseases or conditions should read this book. This drug-free, non-invasive technique is ideal to treat infants, children, grown-ups, old and debilitated people who suffer from mild to severe allergic reactions.

Acknowledgement:

My sincere acknowledgement goes to hundreds of my children (patients) who have received outstanding results through NAET and turned into healthy, productive teenagers now. And I extend my thanks to their parents for believing in me enough to bring them to receive NAET. Without them this book may not have formed.

Foreword:

The foreword is written by a great pediatrician who is also an NAET specialist. He has reproduced the magic of NAET in thousands of young patients in the past few years.

Preface:

In the preface, the author has explained thoroughly one of her patients and her family tree for four generations (all of the family members were the author's patients for years) and their allergic history over a fourteen-year-period. This gives you a clear demonstration of how allergies are handed down to generations after generations through genes and how they can be eliminated permanently or modified successfully through NAET.

Chapter 1: explains the definitions of allergy in various disciplines of medicine and also in laymen's term.

Chapter 2: describes the various categories of allergens and how they affect an allergic person.

Chapter 3: explains Nambudripad's Testing Techniques and gives you information about various allergy testing techniques.

Chapter 4: is a step-by-step method of evaluating your allergic history.

Chapters 5 & 6: commonly seen pediatric allergies and allergy-related illnesses, along with NAET help-tips, suggestions for some helpful supplements including useful home remedies that can be utilized from your kitchen-shelf for quick relief of symptoms are discussed in these chapters.

Chapter 7: demonstrates kinesiological muscle response testing to detect allergies with illustrations and photographs for easier understanding. There are two kinds of reactions: IgE generated and non-IgE generated allergic reactions. In my opinion, non-IgE generated allergic reactions are producing another type of immunoglobulins (probably IgX?) and our laboratories are not equipped to isolate that particular chemical in non-IgE mediated allergic reactions. Kinesiological muscle response testing is sophisticated to recognize such non-IgE mediated reactions as well as IgE mediated reactions. Because of this muscle response testing is the best test to detect allergies.

Chapter 8: examines all 12 major acupuncture meridians and their connections to different parts of the body and brain and how these meridians hold the secret to good health.

Chater 9: shows the reader a few self-help techniques that can help you or your child in an emergency situation.

Chapter 10: discusses the order of NAET treatment protocol. Appropriate case studies along with each NAET allergen gives a better understanding about the effects of allergens in children.

Glossary: the long list of glossary of terms helps the reader understand the description of some unavoidable medical terms used in the book.

Resources: will help you to find the soruces to purchase some of the helpful vitamins, herbs, and other suggested products in the book.

Bibliography: will help you to find the right reading material just in case the reader wants to learn about allergies and allergy-related diseases from NAET and other perspectives.

Index: will help you locate a term or subject faster .

CHAPTER 1

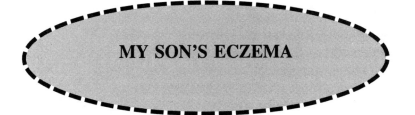

MY SON'S ECZEMA

1

MY SON'S ECZEMA

I *think one of the most devastating childhood diseases is eczema, because I have helplessly watched my children suffering from eczema ever since they were little.*

"Children who suffer from eczema are just parent abusers and need to be on DEMEROL so that their parents can sleep," once said a reportedly knowledgeable dermatologist. Thus began my quest for a solution to relieve my infant son's relentless itching.

An endless stream of visits to allergists and dermatologists proved fruitless. Not one of these respected pediatric physicians was willing to explore the cause of my child's eczema. My reports of skin and breathing difficulties related to oats and peaches, were discounted as being of no consequence. Instead, it was easier to prescribe increasingly stronger topical steroids and oral

3

antihistamines. My frustrations increased as I helplessly watched my young son scratch himself raw. And as his eczema flared, so did his temper. I can only imagine the frustration and discomfort causing his behavioral outbursts.

Four years of searching led me to chiropractic care. We were blessed in that. Dr. Mydlowski was knowledgeable regarding food allergies. A blood sensitivity test uncovered 26 foods that were causing the eczema. At last an answer, but what a blow to normality! Wheat, oats, citrus, dairy, yeast, and peppers to name a few were out of his diet. Parties and snacks at school were difficult, but the day-to- day task of trying to develop tasty, appropriate meals was daunting. The occasional family pizza or dinner out was no longer possible. My four-year-old son was angry, felt punished, not loved, by the dietary limitations. The eczema was improving, but at a psychological cost.

It was then that Dr. Mydlowski heard about NAET. She did not waste any time. She immediately traveled to California and studied NAET and began treating my son using this specially learned medical treatment that utilized the knowledge from acupuncture and oriental medicine but used only acupressure and chiropractic techniques to treat and eliminate allergies permanently. There are no words sufficient to describe the changes that were taking place with this non-invasive, medication-free treatment approach. As each offending food was cleared through NAET, my son's skin cleared up. As the eczema cleared, he became happier. Tantrums decreased from daily to sometimes once per week. Friends and acquaintances began commenting on my son's skin. His hands were not cracked and bleeding. His legs were not rough and red. He was eating pizza and loving it. Within two months my skinny son had gained 3 pounds.

The most astounding elimination of an allergen was to peaches. A taste of peaches at 6 months and 7 months of age and an accidental exposure at 4 years of age had all resulted in trips to the emergency room to treat respiratory distress. There was always the anxiety that a food labeled as containing "natural flavoring" might include peach. For me, treating the peach allergy with NAET was the ultimate test. My son took a taste of peach 25 hours after treatment. I waited anxiously with Benadryl and a nebulizer at hand- no reaction. The next day he ate a half of a peach and by the third day, a whole peach. This fruit is now a regular part of his diet. In fact, I have been able to tell his kindergarten teacher that he can fully participate in cooking projects, and snack time without any restrictions.

Dr. Mydlowski provided not only her expertise and knowledge of NAET, but the emotional support and true interest in my sons as individuals that made our success with the treatment possible. This has been the story of only one of my sons. But I could tell another equally successful story about my other son's freedom from his allergies. Imagine a 13 year old who can go to a friend's house and for the first time not read ingredient labels before eating a snack! We no longer need to bring our own salad dressing to restaurants for fear of MSG triggering an asthmatic attack. There is no grabbing for an "ALBUTEROL" inhaler or leaving church or a restaurant because of someone wearing perfume. The list goes on and on. Most importantly we've become a 'normal' family without the constant fear of exposure to an allergy.

Thank you, NAET.
We love you, Dr. Mydlowski

Debbie O., Columbus, NJ

NAET practitioner: Marybeth Mydlowski, D.C.
861 White House Ave., Hamilton Township, NJ 08610
Tel: (609) 581-8484

Although some medical practitioners may consider allergies as "just an allergy," most clinicians now realize the impact that allergies and allergy-related illnesses have on children's health and how they affect their growth and quality of life.

Epidemiologic survey indicates that the familial trait for allergy is inherited as autosomal recessive. But frequency of positive allergy skin tests is similar in boys and girls.

It is estimated that 90 percent of the population throughout the world suffers from allergies. But the estimate is just that, an estimate, due to the various definitions of allergies among researchers. As already stated, no specific definition for allergy has been universally agreed upon. If medical researchers were willing to broaden their views on allergies to include hypersensitivity, intolerances, IgE- mediated and non-IgE-mediated reactions, we would clearly recognize the overwhelming percentage of allergy sufferers.

Although the medical profession and the public have used the term "allergy" for many decades, knowledge about the nature of allergies, their wide range and implications, is still in an embryonic stage. Even in this enlightened age, many people, including some health professionals, upon hearing the word "allergy" think only of a runny nose, sneezing, hives and perhaps asthma or hay fever. In some instances, the reactions of allergy sufferers are predictable, but for others, the reactions are not at all what would be expected. These reactions vary radically and appear unexpectedly, making diagnosis elusive and pretreatments nearly impossible. Curiously, an increasing number of medical doctors and researchers are now considering that allergic factors may be involved in most illnesses and medical disorders.

According to the statistics released by the American College of Allergy, Asthma and Immunology (ACAAI) in January 1999, approximately 40-50 million Americans have some form of allergy, only one to two percent of all adults are allergic to foods or food additives. Eight percent of children under age six have adverse reactions to ingested foods; only two to five percent have confirmed food allergies.

Without question, there are many undiagnosed allergies hiding beneath the myriad of unresolved health problems inflicted on unsuspecting patients worldwide. The research and experience gathered in my allergy practice confirms that only a fraction of allergies are regularly diagnosed by traditional medical diagnostic measures. Others are missed in diagnostic process since no one has developed a test to isolate the factors or chemical messengers involved in diagnosing sensitivity reactions (mild to severe hypersensitivity). My conclusion is based on 15 years of experience and thousands of case histories not only from my practice, but also from thousands of doctors I have trained in the NAET method. These reactions give the sufferers and their loved ones many anxiety-filled moments, days, and in some cases months or longer. The practitioner may doubt his/her knowledge and ability to practice medicine or get frustrated about the situation and give a scapegoat diagnosis like viral, incurable, genetic, strange, idiopathic and/or psychosomatic. A scapegoat diagnosis gives the patient temporary satisfaction and some momentary peace of mind to the doctor. However, the result is not long lasting to either party.

How Safe Is Our Tap Water To Drink?

Four-year-old Doug had been suffering from severe asthmatic attacks since he was an infant. His mother had tried everything from herbal remedies to conventional allergy specialists. He was given inhalers, steroids, special bedding, air purifiers, and injections to desensitize him to molds, pollens, dust mites, etc., but he ended up in the emergency room at least once a month. He would spend 2-3 hours on an inhaler before his lungs were clear enough for him to breathe by himself. His parents were constantly monitoring him, never wanting to leave him alone. They limited his play time and kept him on a restricted diet. By the time he was brought to the clinic, Doug was pale, weak and had so much difficulty breathing that he was using his facial muscles to help him breathe. I listened to his lungs through a stethoscope and they were totally filled with liquid. When I let his mother listen she grew pale. After muscle testing, he was found to be allergic to the chemicals in the water he was drinking daily. After treating him for the chemicals in drinking water I let his mother listen to his chest again. His lungs were perfectly clear! He hasn't had any difficulty breathing since. He plays, eats, drinks and looks as healthy as all his friends at his preschool now.

Any of the allergens can trigger various allergic responses in sensitive individuals. Most of the allergic diseases are immuno-globulin E (IgE) mediated immunologic illnesses that affect the person's organ systems either individually or collectively. Nonimmune reactions may be caused by the interactions of the allergen's physical or chemical properties with the plasma protein of the host causing to release substances like cytokines, histamines, etc. It seems currently available laboratory tests are not very sensitive in registering the pathways of production of such chemical messengers that are responsible in producing various types and degrees of nonimmune allergic reactions we see in our patients everyday. So we are forced to limit our understanding of the allergic reactions as IgE-mediated and non-IgE-mediated. As of now, non-IgE mediated reactions are not called allergies by traditional medical researchers because they cannot yet identify or isolate the pathway for creating such reactions. Since no immunoglobulins or chemical messengers are identified, these reactions are named as simple hypersensitivity reactions or intolerances.

Whether it is an IgE-mediated or non-IgE-mediated reaction, it is obvious that many people are affected by the impact of this disorder in varying degrees ranging from mild to severe. Because of these food intolerances and hypersensitivity reactions many children spend their important childhood in the doctors' offices instead of school classrooms, grow up unhealthy due to malabsorption of the nutrients and end up as sickly adults. If we could develop more sensitive laboratory tests, we would have a definitive answer to various reactions our children suffer in their daily life. If we could find the cause we could find a proper cure which could produce a healthy population.

An allergy can be defined as an attack of a person's body against its own immune system (the body's defense system), when it comes in contact with any substance to which it reacts adversely, even though that substance may be, in reality, harmless or even useful to the body.

This spontaneous, severe reaction of the immune system towards the suspected allergen produces a particular immunoglobulin (IgE in most cases), when the body is exposed to what it thinks is a foreign and dangerous substance. These immunoglobulins (antibodies) react with allergens to release "histamines" or other chemicals from the cells that produce different allergic symptoms.

A normal immune system will immediately release substances that are more appropriate to fight the unexpected reactions.

Some of these substances include: corticosteroids, cortisone, heparin, prostaglandins, endorphins, enkephalin, neurokinins, interleukins, interferons, antihistamines, cytokines, adrenaline, that are appropriate to the specific condition to counteract the allergic reactions. Then the body will come to a settlement with the allergen in seconds without causing any obvious ill-health symptoms in the person. But when the immune system perceives what should be harmless substances as dangerous intruders and stimulates antibody production to defend the body, things do not settle down as pleasantly as in the person with a normal immune system.

Here, the first contact with an allergen initiates the baby step of an allergic reaction inside the body. The body will alert its defense forces in response to the alarm received about the new invader and will immediately produce a few antibodies, storing them in reserve for future use.

In most people, a first contact or initial sensitization will usually not produce many symptoms. During the second exposure to the allergen, the body will alert the previously produced antibodies to action, producing more noticeable symptoms.

If you have a normal or a fairly strong immune system, you may not get severe reactions even with the second exposure. But often with the third exposure, the threatened immune system will begin serious action causing allergic reactions in the body.

Usually IgE - is the antibody that is responsible for immediate allergic reactions in the body when it comes in contact with an allergen. There are other types of immunoglobulins produced in the body at various instances as a natural defense mechanism to protect the body. Some of the known ones include:

IgA - is produced when the reactions are associated with the mucous membranes.
IgD - is found on the surface of the B-cells.

IgG - is also known as gamma globulin, which produces a delayed reaction, with symptoms taking anywhere from a few hours to 3 - 4 days to appear. IgG is the major antibody in the blood that protects against bacteria and viruses.

IgM - is the first antibody to appear during an immune response.

IgX - is the chemical messenger probably responsible for nonimmune reactions in the body causing intolerances and mild to severe form of hypersensitivity reactions, but this one is yet to be discovered in the coming years.

An allergic reaction may be manifested in varying degrees as mild to severe itching, rashes, hives or swelling anywhere within the body. The most commonly affected areas are the skin, eyes, nose, throat, lungs, mouth, rectum and vaginal mucosa.

Even though allergic diseases and reactions usually are not fatal, sometimes these reactions can cause major concerns regarding the health of the sufferer. Death can also result from certain allergic reactions especially if there is an anaphylactic reaction to the allergen. Allergies are known to cause anaphylaxis in very sensitive individuals. The known allergens causing anaphylactic reactions belong to these groups: related to foods (shellfish, peanut, MSG -also known as monosodium glutamate), medications and hospital procedures (penicillin, aspirin, vaccines, blood transfusions, plasma transfusions, organ transplants, graft-versus- host diseases), venom from an insect or insect stings (bee, wasp, spider), environmental pollutants and chemicals (paint, chemical fumes, formaldehyde, pesticides, hair dye, etc.). Anaphylaxis is a systemic generalized allergic response consisting of number of symptoms. An anaphylactic shock can affect a few or all organs at the same time, giving rise to exaggerated systemic symptoms, manifesting in sharp pains in the head, abdomen and chest. It can also cause swelling of the tongue and throat leading to constriction and breathing difficulties, or a partial shutdown of blood circulation causing low blood pressure, fast heart rate and thready pulse or no pulse at all. Additional symptoms we've seen include decrease in body temperature leading to cold and clammy skin, sensation of chills, internal cold, pallor, rolling eyes, sensation of fear, fever, unresponsiveness, light-headedness, nausea, diarrhea, panic attack, fainting, and at times, even death due to complete shut down of the system.

Children are affected by various allergies in everyday life. Their immune system is not fully ready to fight the pathogens and adverse reactions they face in everyday-life. If they have a poor immune system, boosting up the immune system is essential to maintaining good health. Some of the most common childhood disorders arising from allergies are discussed in the following pages.

Bronchopulmonary reactions like upper respiratory disorders and asthma are major chronic illnesses among children in United States and usually they develop from some kind of allergies. Asthma is the ninth leading cause of hospitalization nationally. It is one of the leading causes of school absenteeism in children in this country. The allergic tendency toward asthma is often inherited. Asthma is twice as common in males as in females prior to adolescence, but appears equal in prevalence thereafter. According to the statistics released from CDC, approximately 50 million people in the U. S. A. suffer from asthma. It is estimated that the heath care cost for asthma alone is more than 6.2 billion dollars in the U. S. A. annually.

Of the IgE-mediated allergies, allergic rhinitis is the most prevalent disorder of childhood affecting 15% of all children. The triggers for this disorder may be hidden as an allergy to the dust, dust mites, pollens, grasses, flowers, perfumes, smell from plastic toys, crib-toys, fungus, molds, synthetic fabrics, detergents, stuffed toys, pets and animals. Refined starches and sugars also produce symptoms of allergic rhinitis, especially in children.

Gastrointestinal allergy is most often associated with food allergy; however, foods also can cause allergic reactions in other systems: fever, fatigue, eczema, shortness of breath, restlessness, insomnia, autism, attention deficit and/or hyperactive disorders, learning disability, dyslexia, behavioral disorders and many other psychological disorders.

According to the 1998 statement by the National Institutes of Health, an estimated 3% to 5% of school age children are suffering from ADHD, making it the most commonly diagnosed behavioral disorder of childhood.

ADHD was thought to be exclusively a childhood disease that required only temporary medication. But, the latest research has shown that 50% of children with ADHD may carry the disorder into adulthood and become ADHD adults.

If we carefully evaluate these children with different disorders we could find out that these children are in fact suffering from allergies, hypersensitivities or food intolerances. They could be allergic to everyday food groups: milk, eggs, breads, cereals, juices, fruits, or the school materials: books, coloring agents, play dough, or pens or pencils. The focus of this book will emphasize how to uncover the causes of some of these commonly seen childhood disorders brought on by above mentioned simple allergens that cause the children to have the disabilities in sequencing, abstraction, organization, memory, language, and motor skills.

If the allergen could be uncovered and isolated, if they were eliminated as they are detected, these children wouldn't have to suffer the unpleasantness through their childhood and carry the burden into their adulthood. How can you do that?

Read on to explore the answer for yourself!

When we look at an allergy from a holistic point of view, we can say that an allergy is an energy imbalance caused by the clashing of two or more incompatible energies. This is similar to like-magnetic charges repelling one another with a slight difference. The repulsion of the incompatible energies cause an allergic reaction, an altered action in the body.

Hundreds of researchers, doctors, and scientifically oriented patients ask me the same question: "Are you treating real allergies or just treating intolerances and sensitivities?" The symptoms, diagnosis and treatments of sensitivities, hypersensitivities and intolerances, (non-IgE mediated reactions) and allergies (IgE mediated reactions) often overlap. Both intolerances and allergies, in varying degrees, can be tested by Muscle Response Testing (MRT) either by producing a weak MRT (weakness of the indicator muscle in the case of an allergy), or strong MRT (strong resistance by the indicator muscle in the case where there is no allergy). All of these allergic reactions can successfully be treated by NAET. MRT and NAET are explained in detail in Chapter 7.

Even though we have a few sophisticated, scientifically oriented diagnostic tests available, western medicine still has no clear answers as to why various health disorders happen the way they do. On the other hand, oriental medicine through its unsophisticated simple testing and evaluating procedures demonstrate the reasons for many sicknesses in young and old. When we understand the oriental medical procedures and try to follow their treatment plans we can see outstanding results in the sufferers.

Proof is in the Pudding!

According to oriental medical principles, the Yin-Yang balanced state represents the perfect balance of energies. Any imbalance in a Yin-Yang state causes an energy difference. Yin-Yang does not represent an item. It is a term used to compare the state of two energies in or around us. Any imbalance in the Yin-Yang state causes disharmony. We can find various types and kinds of energy imbalances not only in many aspects of a person's life, but also between two items.

Is there a Relationship between Allergy and common childhood disorders?

In my NAET allergy practice, I have found working with children and their parents to be challenging. But, by treating the children with NAET, I have been able to receive a great amount of satisfaction and success in dealing with common everyday ailments of little children. I have treated many hundreds of young children from different age groups who were diagnosed as suffering from various disorders including attention deficit hyperactive disorders. One group was clearly diagnosed by appropriate medical practitioners and their diagnosis was supported by various tests. The other group never had any concise diagnosis, yet suffered from the typical symptoms. In both groups, normal living was difficult until they were treated with NAET.

When I examined the children using NTT (Nambudripad's Testing Techniques), regardless of the labels they carry, I found these children suffered from various food and environmental allergies. When I treated them with NAET (Nambudripad's Allergy Elimination Techniques), children responded very well making it possible to eliminate their symptoms and live a normal life.

If the practitioner is not well informed about allergies and allergy-related symptoms, it is easy to misdiagnose allergy-related illnesses.

In this book, I am going to demonstrate how allergy to foods, environments, childhood immunizations, vaccinations, lacking certain internal body secretions, or producing abnormal enzymes, can generate, complicate or exaggerate the symptoms of various childhood health disorders. You will learn about a simple testing procedure that will enable you to test your child in the privacy of your own home using NAET, the procedure that can help to remove allergies and allergy related diseases. I will describe some techniques that can help to improve your child's overall health and balance the body and mind during the journey through NAET. But I would like you to understand one thing: that NAET is not magic; it is hard work. The hard work that will pay you great dividends given enough time!

An allergy is a hereditary condition: an allergic predisposition or tendency is inherited, but the allergy itself may not manifest until some later date. Researchers have found that when both parents were or are allergy-sensitive, 75 to 100 percent of their offspring react to those same allergens. When neither of the parents is (nor was) sensitive to allergens, the probability of producing allergic offspring drops dramatically to less than 10 percent. Most of us suffer from allergic manifestation in varying degrees because of our different levels of parental inheritance.

Studies have shown that, in some cases, even when parents had no allergies, their offspring still suffered from many allergies since birth. In these cases, various possibilities exist:

•   Parents may have suffered from a serious disease or condition. For example, the parents had rheumatic fever before the child was born, which caused an alteration in the genetic codes.

• The pregnant mother may have been exposed to harmful substances such as radiation (X-rays); chemicals (an expectant mother taking too much caffeine, alcohol, drugs or antibiotics, chemical exposures, carbon monoxide poisoning, etc.); circulating internal toxins as the result of a disease (streptococcal infection as in strep-throat, measles, chicken pox, candidiasis, parasitic infestation, diabetes, etc.); emotional trauma (sudden loss of loved ones, various kinds of abuses like mental torture, rapes, fearful falls, financial struggles, traumatic law suits, continuous harassment by others, etc.).

• The parents may have suffered severe malnutrition (not getting enough food or not assimilating due to poor absorption or allergies) possibly causing the growing embryo to undergo cell mutation during its development in the womb. The altered cells do not carry over the original genetic codes or do not go through normal development. The organs and tissues that are supposed to develop from the affected cells have impaired function.

• In our modern day life, many parents leave their infants in front of the color television permitting the infant to bathe in continuous flow of radiation for hours. Excess assimilation of television radiation can cause energy blockages and cell mutation in the growing infant.

We cannot ignore the fact that we are moving toward the twenty-first century where technology will be even more predominant than today. There is nothing wrong with the technology, but the allergic patient must find ways to overcome adverse reactions to chemicals and other allergens, in order to live a better life.

What Is NAET?

A thorough treatise on biochemistry is not appropriate for the purpose of an introduction to this new method of treatment for people suffering from allergies. Instead, this discussion will concentrate on the basic constructs of this treatment method and give some insight into the lives of people that it has helped. This is not a new technology. It is actually a combination of knowledge and techniques that uses much of what is already known from allopathic (western medical knowledge), chiropractic, kinesiology, acupuncture (oriental medical knowledge) and nutrition. Each of the disciplines I studied provided bits of knowledge, which I used to develop this new allergy elimination treatment. There is no known successful method of treatment for food allergies using western medicine except avoidance, which means deprivation and frustration.

I developed this new technique of allergy and allergy-related symptom elimination, employing the knowledge from these above mentioned fields of medicine, to identify and treat for the reactions to many substances, including food, chemicals, and environmental allergens.

Through many long years of research, and after many trials and errors, I devised this combination of "hands-on techniques" to eliminate energy blockages (allergies) permanently and to restore the body to a healthy state. These energy blockage elimination techniques together are called Nambudripad's Allergy Elimination Techniques or NAET for short.

Allopathy And Western Science

Knowledge of the brain, cranial nerves, spinal nerves and autonomic nervous system from western medicine enlightens us about the body's efficient multilevel communication network. Through this network of nerves, vital energy circulates in the body carrying negative and positive messages from each and every cell to the brain and then back to the cells. A cell or tissue sends one message to brain. The brain sends out the reply in a matter of nanoseconds to the rest of the body. Knowledge about the nervous system, its origin, travel route, organs and tissues that benefit from its nerve energy supply (target organs and tissues), helps us to understand the energy distribution of the spinal nerves emerging from the 31 pairs of spinal nerve roots. If the energy supply reaches all the respective organs and tissues, through their miles-long nerve fibers, they all remain healthy and happy. If the energy distribution is reduced or stopped in one or more of the spinal nerves, the respective organs and tissues will have diminished function or partial or complete shut down. By evaluating the condition of its target organs and tissues, changes in energy distribution via any spinal nerve can be detected (Gray's Anatomy-36th edition).

Kinesiology

Kinesiology is the art and science of movement of the human body. Kinesiology is used in NAET to compare the strength and weakness of any muscle of the body in the presence or absence of any substance. This is also called Muscle Response Testing to detect allergies. It is hypothesized that this measurable weakness of a particular muscle is produced by the generation of an energy obstruction in the particular spinal nerve route that corresponds to the weakened muscle when the specific item is in its energy field. Any item that is capable of producing energy obstruction in any spinal nerve root is called an allergen. Through this simple kinesiological testing method allergens can be detected; obstructed spinal nerves and their routes can be identified; and the affected organs, tissues, and other body parts can be uncovered.

Pilot Study On Muscle Response Testing

Muscle testing to detect allergies is supported by the pilot study done by Walter H. Schmitt Jr. and Gerry Leisman, "Applied Neuro Science Laboratories," N.C., U.S.A., and the College of Judea and Samaria, P.O. Box 3, Arie, 44837, Israel, titled CORRE-

LATION OF APPLIED KINESIOLOGY MUSCLE TESING FINDINGS WITH SERUM IMMUNOGLOBULIN LEVELS FOR FOOD ALLERGY, AUGUST 1998.

Chiropractic

Chiropractic technique helps us to detect the nerve energy blockage in a specific nerve energy pathway by detecting and isolating the exact nerve root that is being pinched. The exact vertebral level in relation to the pinched spinal nerve root helps us to trace the travel route, the destination and the target organs of that particular energy pathway. D.D. Palmer, who is considered the "Father of Chiropractic" said, "too much or too little energy is disease." According to chiropractic theory, a pinched nerve can cause disturbance in the energy flow. Earlier we saw that the presence of an allergen in one's energy field can cause a pinched nerve or obstruction of the nerve energy flow. Chiropractic medicine postulates that a pinched nerve or any such disturbance in the energy flow can cause disease in the target organ and tissues, revealing the importance of maintaining an uninterrupted flow of nerve energy. A pinched nerve or an obstruction in the energy flow can result from an allergy. Spinal manipulation at the specific vertebral level of the pinched nerve can relieve the obstruction of the energy flow and help the body come to a state of homeostasis (i.e. a state of perfect balance between all energies and functions).

Acupuncture/ Oriental Medicine

Yin-Yang theory from oriental medical principles also teaches the importance of maintaining homeostasis in the body. According to oriental medical principles, "when the Yin and Yang are balanced in the body (a state of perfect balance between all energies and functions), no disease is possible." Any disturbance in the homeostasis can cause disease. Any allergen that is capable of producing a weakening effect of the muscles in the body can cause disturbance in the homeostasis. By isolating and eliminating the cause of the disturbance (in this case an allergen), and by maintaining an absolute homeostasis, diseases can be prevented and cured. According to acupuncture theory, acupuncture and/or acupressure at certain acupuncture points are capable of bringing the body into a state of homeostasis, by removing the energy blockages from the twelve (meridian) energy pathways. When the blockages are removed, energy can flow freely through the energy meridians bringing the body into perfect balance.

Nutrition

You are what you eat! The secret to good health is achieved through correct nutrition. What is correct nutrition? How do you get it? When you can eat nutritious food without discomfort and assimilate the nutrients from the food, that food is the right food. When you get indigestion, bloating, and other digestive troubles upon or after eating a particular food, that food is not helping you to function normally. However natural, expensive or packed with high quality nutrition, if a food item causes one or more of these symptoms upon ingestion, it is not the right nutrition for you. This is due to an allergy to that food. Different people react differently to the same food. So, it is very important to clear the allergy to the nutrients, which are in the food. Allergic people can tolerate food that is low in nutrition better than nutritious food. After clearing the allergy, you should try to eat more wholesome, nutritious foods. Above all, you should avoid refined, bleached food devoid of nutrients.

Many people who feel poorly due to undiagnosed food allergies may take vitamins or other supplements to increase their vitality. This can actually make them feel worse if they happen to be allergic to these nutrients as well. Only after clearing those allergies can their bodies properly assimilate them. So nutritional assessment should be done periodically, and if needed, appropriate supplements should be taken to receive better results.

We need the complete cooperation of the whole brain and nervous system to get the best results with NAET. NAET involves the whole brain and its network of nerves, as it reprograms the brain by erasing previously harmful memory regarding the allergen and imprints the new useful memory in its place.

Imbalances

The energy blockages in the human body are caused by incompatible electromagnetic charges around the body. When there is an incompatible charge around the body, there is an altered reaction in the body. Energy incompatibilities that are capable of producing various ailments are used synonymously with "allergy" in this book.

When we talk about health conditions, there is hardly a human disease or condition that may not involve an allergic factor. Any portion of the body, organ, or group of organs may be involved with a particular allergy, though the allergic responses may vary greatly from one item to another and from one person to another.

In 1983, I originated NAET to eliminate allergic reactions and successfully restore normal functions of the body by manipulating the spinal nerves. Major illnesses, severe reactions to drugs, toxins, chemicals, radiation, emotional stresses, etc., are capable of causing damage to the sensory nerve fibers and inhibiting their conductivity. Allergy and allergy-related illnesses can thus be eliminated or reduced in their intensity by treating with NAET.

The brain, through 31 pairs of spinal nerves, operates the best network of communication ever known. Energy blockages take place in a person's body due to contact with adverse energy of other substances. When two adverse energies come close, repulsion takes place. When two compatible energies get together, attraction takes place.

NAET can unblock the blockages in the energy pathways and restart normal energy circulation through the energy channels. This will, in turn, help the brain to work and coordinate with the rest of the body to operate the body functions appropriately. When the brain is not coordinating with the vital organs, physiological functions are impaired.

When the energy circulation in the energy pathways is restored, the vital organs resume their routine work and function properly. The brain and body together will remove any toxic buildup through the body's natural excretory mechanisms.

When the energy channels are filled with vibrant energy, and the energy circulates through the channels freely, the body is said to be in perfect balance or in homeostasis. When the body is in homeostasis, it can function normally, and allergies and diseases do not affect the body. In this state, the body can absorb all the necessary nutrients from the foods consumed.

The energy channels need energy to function normally. This energy is produced from the nutrients consumed, such as vitamins, minerals, and sugars, etc. The attraction or repulsion of the electromagnetic energy field is created in the body by the interaction of the various charged nutrients inside the body. Each cell is an electricity-generating unit loaded with positively charged potassium and some sodium. Most of the sodium is outside the cell. The sodium and potassium keep circulating in and out of the cell in the presence of water with the help of other nutrients like proteins and sugars. These charged molecules inside the body make the whole body an electrical unit with an electrical field around it.

These nearly 90% effective, successful NAET treatments are available to the whole world. It is up to the health professionals to learn them and use them on their patients, and it is up to the public to get them from their doctors to receive full benefits of this new, remarkably effective treatment method.

Thousands of doctors of allopathic, chiropractic, osteopathy, dentistry, naturopathy, and acupuncture/oriental medicine from all over the United States, Canada, Europe, Australia, Asia and other countries, have been trained to treat their patients with this new revolutionary technique. Regular training sessions are being conducted several times a year to prepare many more licensed medical professionals to meet the challenge. This book will educate individuals to test themselves and locate the cause of their problem. Steps of treatments are not given here, because that is beyond the scope of this book. The information about the NAET training available for licensed medical practitioners can be received from the following sources:

NAET
6714 Beach Blvd.
Buena Park, CA 90621
Tel: 714-523-8900 / (714) 523 0800
Fax: 714-523-3068
E-mail: naet@earthlink.net
Web site: www.naet.com

CHAPTER 2

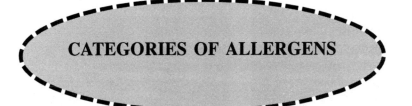

CATEGORIES OF ALLERGENS

2

Categories Of Allergens

Peanut Anaphylaxis

*S*ince NAET has helped my son, C.J. {Charles Jr.} in *so many ways, I don't know where to begin this story. I like to shout at the whole world, to the desperate mothers not finding the right help for their sick children, please don't get discouraged, don't give up, there is real help out there for you and for your child--- find NAET. It is simple, painless, drugless, all natural, to help your child overcome most of his/her health problems. NAET changed my son's life, and my life, and our lives. It can change your child's life ---and your life too.*

My son was deathly allergic to peanuts. As well, he also had moderate asthma, numerous food, chemical, and environmental allergies.

When he was a baby he suffered colic for many months. He often cried for hours on end, and at times was not consolable in any capacity. At about 1 year old I decided there had to be something doctors could do other than what had already been suggested. I went to 5 different pediatricians searching for help. Not once was allergies even suggested. Now this was 10 years ago. and I, myself had no understanding of how allergies could have such an effect on an individual. As he grew into a toddler, he became a difficult child. He would throw long fits, and it was as though he was possessed or something. The incident would suddenly come to a halt and he would be fine again. He had begun to get violent with hitting, scratching, and biting. I was very worried about what would become of him.

In addition he had by now been hospitalized a few times for asthma attacks, and been in the emergency room about 4 times for peanut allergy reactions. Two of these were anaphylactic shock reactions.

In the summer of 1997 I found a Natural Health magazine, and the front cover said "A food Allergy Cure You Won't Believe". I read it, and though very skeptical, went to the internet and found only 4 doctors listed for Illinois, of which Dr. Pamela Olson was one! I had just had allergy testing done a couple of months previous to this, and found by skin test that I had numerous allergies, and thought at that point this was probably the root of my son's problems.

I went to Dr. Olson first, to see if this was going to work, and make sure it would not be dangerous to my son. The results were fabulous, and I knew we were on to something wonderful!

He started NAET that October, and after clearing many allergies to numerous foods, chemicals, and all environmental allergies we decided to try the nuts. It took several different clearings, but in the end, with the guidance of Dr. Olson and Dr. Devi, my son is now completely free of his peanut allergy! His asthma has diminished by about 85%. If we have any problem with it, we just go see Dr. Olson! No more steroids!

We never had a rast test done. His pediatrician refused to do the test, and I didn't want the added expense and explanation as to why we needed the test done, since he had no other treatments done by any other doctor. I know from what he now eats that he is completely rid of the allergy. I often remind him that I would still like to know if he wants to eat something containing peanuts just to be on the safe side! I don't think the old fear has left me all the way.

Incidentally, He is no longer violent. He has no more fits of rage. He is happy, healthy, and well adjusted! He is friendly, cooperative, and a straight A student in school.

NAET has changed our lives in so many ways. I still get tears in my eyes when I think of what Dr. Devi's technique has done for my family. I will never be able to thank her enough for this God sent gift she has brought to all of us.

Yours Sincerely,
Terri J. Preucil
Charles Kaskadden Jr.

Classification of Allergens

Commonly seen allergens are generally classified into nine basic categories; based primarily on the method in which they are contacted, rather than the symptoms they produce.

1. Inhalants
2. Ingestants
3. Contactants
4. Injectants
5. Infectants
6. Physical Agents
7. Genetic Factors
8. Molds and Fungi
9. Emotional Factors

Inhalants

Inhalants are those allergens that are contacted through the nose, throat and bronchial tubes. Examples of inhalants are microscopic spores of certain grasses, flowers, pollens, powders, smoke, cosmetics, perfumes, different aromas from spices, coffee, popcorn, food-cooking smells, different herbs and oils and chemical fumes such as paint, varnish, pesticides, insecticides, fertilizers, and flour from grains, etc.

It is typical for a sensitive person to react to most of these environmental allergens. The symptoms arising from the interactions with the above allergens, varies greatly from patient to patient.

Ingestants

Ingestants are allergens, which are contacted through the mouth and find their way into the gastrointestinal tract. These include foods, condiments, drugs, beverages, chewing gum, and vitamin supplements, etc. We must not ignore the potential reactions to things that are touched, then inadvertently transmitted into the mouth through our hands.

The area of ingested allergens is one of the most difficult to diagnose because the allergic responses are often delayed from several minutes to several days. This makes the direct association between cause and effect very difficult. Some people can react violently in seconds after they consume an allergen. In extreme cases, just touching or coming near the allergen is enough to forewarn the central nervous system that it is about to be poisoned resulting in a premature allergic reaction. Usually more violent reactions are observed in ingested allergens.

Such was the case of eight-year-old Don, who complained of having a stomach ache every day for six months. He became very irritable at times. His parents noticed how his personality was changing. He was becoming antisocial, refusing to go out and play with other children. He stayed home when he was not in school. He did not do his schoolwork or homework and began to get poor grades. His teacher reported that he was turning into a loner. His parents were called to the school many times because of his problems. They took Don to the pediatrician, after administering a battery of tests, he was diagnosed as having ADHD.

One of his mother's friends, whose son was successfully treated by me for celiac disease, had similar symptoms and behavioral problems initially. He became normal when the celiac disease was under control by treating with NAET. She referred him to us. Don was examined by NTT, and found to be allergic to 18 basic groups of foods from the NAET list. His treatments were very successful until he reached the grain mix. He failed grain mix three times. He was highly allergic to the wheat and gluten in the mix, which caused him to fail the treatment. His strange behavior and stomach ache was under control when he passed the treatment for grain mix.

We live in a highly technological age. New substances are being introduced into our diets to preserve color, flavor, and extend the shelf life of our foods. There are some additives used in foods as preservatives that have caused severe health problems. Some artificial sweeteners cause mysterious problems in particular people. They may mimic symptoms of serious disorders (ADD, hyperactivity, autism, and behavioral problems, etc.). Clinical depression, antisocial behaviors, itching and hives, insomnia, vertigo, are also reactions from an allergy to food coloring and preservatives. The majority of these additives are harmless to most people but can be disabling and life-threatening to those who react to these substances.

Great care must be taken to know exactly what is contained in anything a person with allergies puts into his mouth. If everyone could become proficient in MRT, simple testing before eating foods could prevent most hazardous reactions from food allergies.

Contactants

Contactants produce their effect by direct contact with the skin. They include environmental allergens, fabrics, cats, dogs, rabbits, cosmetics, soaps, skin creams, detergents, rubbing alcohol, latex gloves, hair dyes, various types of plant oils, and chemicals such as gasoline, dyes, acrylic nails, nail polish, fabrics, form-aldehyde, etc.

Allergic reactions to contactants can be different in each person, and may produce any commonly seen health disorders. Various natural or synthetic fabrics can cause allergic reactions in children. Many people react to cotton. Cotton is used in numerous items. It is not easy to find a fabric that is made from only one type of material anymore. Many products seen in shops are a blend of many things. Cotton fibers are used in carpets, elastics, bed sheet, fleece material, cosmetic applicators, toilet paper, paper towels, etc. Wool may also cause reactions in sensitive persons. Some people who are sensitive to wool also react to creams with a lanolin base since lanolin is derived from sheep wool. Some people can be allergic to cotton socks, nylon socks or woolen socks, causing them to have abnormal and irrational behaviors. People can also be allergic to carpets and drapes that can cause similar reactions in sensitive individuals.

Usually, female patients are allergic to their pantyhose and suffer from leg cramps, swollen legs, high blood pressure, headaches, mood swings and crying spells. Toilet paper and paper towels also cause problems mimicking similar reactions in many people.

A lot of people are allergic to crude oils, plant oils and their derivatives, which include plastic and synthetic rubber products as well as latex products. Can you imagine the difficulty of living in this modern society, attempting to be completely free from products made of crude oil? A person would literally be immobilized. The phones we use, the milk containers we drink from, the polyester fabrics we wear, most of the face and body creams we use... all are made from a common product – crude oil!

Food items normally classified as ingestants—may also act as contactants on persons who handle them constantly over time. They can cause migraines, headaches, brain irritability, anger, and depression, etc.

Other career-produced allergies have been diagnosed in cooks, waiters, grocery storekeepers, clerks, gardeners, etc.

Virtually no trade or skill is exempt from contacting allergens and producing allergic symptoms.

A writer by profession, Nelly was completely disabled with her nervous stomach, irritable bowel syndrome, insomnia, and heart palpitations. She was easily angered and had sinusitis and postnasal drip for seven years. She was given an NTT evaluation and it was found that she was allergic to newspaper ink and all kinds of paper including toilet paper, and dollar bills. Nelly was simply allergic to the paper she wrote on. Her symptoms started seven years ago, not long after she began her career as a writer. After she was treated for all the NAET basics and the paper products by NAET, her symptoms cleared.

Another case of a paper allergy was observed during an interview with an attorney who complained that he always came away from his office with a severe headache. His personality would change and he would become hostile and angry at the least little thing. His family would hide in another room not to be in his way. The attorney was allergic to paper—but his reaction was completely different from that of the professional writer.

Injectant

Allergens are injected into the skin, muscles, joints and blood vessels in the form of various serums, antitoxins, vaccines, childhood immunizations, and drugs. Injectant also include substances entering the body through insect bites. As with any other allergic reaction, the injection of a sensitive drug into the system creates the risk of producing dangerous allergic reactions. To the sensitive person, the drug actively becomes a poison with the same effect as an injection of arsenic. The seemingly harmless substance can become more allergenic for certain people over time without the person being aware of the potential risk. For example, take the increasing number of incidents of allergies to the drug penicillin. The reactions vary from hives to diarrhea to anaphylactic shock and death.

Various vaccinations and immunizations may also produce such allergic reactions. After receiving their usual immunizations, some children become extremely ill physically, physiologically, and emotionally. Various neurological disorders, hyperactive disorders, attention deficit disorders, autism, mental retardation, manic disorders, Crohn's disease, chronic irritable bowel syndrome, tumors, and cysts, etc., could manifest as a delayed reaction of a childhood immunization.

Such was the case of a 6-year-old boy David, who became very sick after a regular DPT immunization. He had a continuous fever (102 degrees Fahrenheit) that lasted for six weeks. Finally, when the fever came down to a normal level, he became irritable, aggressive, short tempered, antisocial. He couldn't play with other children without kicking, hitting, biting or spitting on them. He talked constantly and craved sweets all the time. He ran around the house playing hide and seek in the middle of the night instead of sleeping. His worried parents brought him to see me. His problem was traced to the DPT immunization by testing using NTT. He was treated for all the basics and DPT vaccine with NAET. He became well again after he was treated for DPT.

Infectants

Infectants are allergens that produce their effect by causing sensitivity to an infectious agent, such as bacteria. For example, an allergic reaction may result when tuberculin bacterium is introduced as part of a diagnostic test to determine a patient's sensitivity or reaction to it. A typical reaction to the tuberculin test may be seen as an infectious eruption under the skin. This type of reaction may occur with a skin patch or scratch tests performed in the normal course of allergy testing in traditional medical approach.

Infectants differ from injectants because of the nature of the allergic substance; that is a substance, which is a known injectant and is limited in the amount administered to the patient. A slight prick of the skin introduces the toxin through the epidermis and a pox, or similar harmless skin lesion will erupt if the patient is allergic to that substance. For most people, the pox soon dries up and forms a scab that eventually heals, without much discomfort. However, in some cases the site of the injectant becomes infected and the usual inflammatory process can be seen (redness, swelling, pain, drainage of pus from the site for many days). Some sensitive individuals may experience fainting, nausea, fever, swelling (not only at the scratch site but also over the whole body), and respiratory distress, etc., if left untreated.

In other words, the introduction of an allergen into a reactive person's system creates the potential risk of causing a severe response regardless of the amount of the toxic substance used. Great care must be taken in the administration of traditional allergy testing procedures in highly sensitive individuals. However, if NAET is administered correctly and immediately it can stop such adverse reactions.

Teresa, a 31-year-old female born in one of the developing countries, was one of our unique cases. She manifested tremendous allergic reactions to a multitude of foods and objects in the environment. Her history revealed that when she was two-years-old, she suffered a severe reaction after a routine BCG vaccination. Her left hand swelled and she suffered from a high fever for weeks. She almost died from the infection. Medical help was not readily available in the part of the country where she grew up. Her parents migrated to the United States when she was seven-years-old. For many years she suffered physical allergies such as asthma, hives, joint pains, migraines, and gastrointestinal allergies (indigestion, heartburn, intermittent chronic diarrhea or constipation), and emotional reactions (depression, anger, crying spells, lacking interest in day-to-day activities, and severe premenstrual syndrome, etc.). When she was treated for all the basics, smallpox vaccination and bacteria mix by NAET, she was able to clear her allergic reactions to various items. Her physical, physiological, and emotional symptoms improved and stabilized swiftly after the treatment.

It should be noted that bacteria and virus are contacted in numerous ways. Our casual contact with objects and people exposes us daily to dangerous contaminants and possible illnesses. When our autoimmune systems are functioning properly, we pass off the illness without notice. It is when our systems are not working at maximum performance levels that we experience infections, fevers, and other discomforts.

From a strictly allergenic standpoint, however, contact with an injectant does not always produce the expected reaction. The intensity and type of reactions vary from individual to individual depending on their immune system, age and the amount of injectant received.

Physical Agents

Heat, humid air, cold, cold mist, sun radiation, dampness, drafts, changes in barometric pressure, high altitude, air conditioning; other types of radiation like computer, microwave, X-ray, geopathic radiation, electrical and electromagnetic radiation, fluorescent lights, radiation from cellular and cordless telephones, and radiation from power lines are irritants. Vibrations from a washer and dryer, hair dryer, electric shaver, massager, motion vibrations from a moving automobile, motion sickness (car sickness, sea sickness), sickness while playing sports, roller coaster rides and/or horseback riding are mechanical irritants. Airplane sounds, traffic noises, loud music and voices in a particular pitch may also cause allergic reactions. All the above are known as physical allergens. Burns may also be included in this category.

When the patient suffers from more than one allergy, physical agents can affect the patient greatly. If the patient has already eaten an allergic food item, then walks in cold air, he might develop upper respiratory problems, a sore throat, asthma or joint pains, etc., depending on his/her tendency toward particular health problems.

It is not uncommon for children to suffer from repeated canker sores. They suffer from sluggish digestion due to many food allergies, and food remains longer in the small bowel. According to oriental medical principles, when food remains in the small bowel too long, the undigested food produces a large amount of heat. The heat escapes through the mouth causing the delicate mucous membrane of the mouth to blister and form canker sores. One of the young patients, Alan who came to our office had a history of canker sores whenever he ate pizza for dinner. He turned out to be highly allergic to tomato sauce (spices and tomato). After the basics, he was treated for tomato mix and pepper mix. He has never been bothered by canker sores again.

Many symptoms like asthma, etc., become exaggerated on cold, cloudy or rainy days. The patients could suffer from a severe allergy to carbon dioxide (their own breath), electrolytes, cold or a combination of all. Some people, especially people who suffer from mental imbalances, also react to moonlight or moon radiation.

Some young patients experience irritability, fear, and anxiety attacks when taking a hot shower. They are also allergic to humidity and can be successfully treated with NAET. A glass jar with a lid is filled half way with hot water. An NAET practitioner administers the NAET treatment while the patient holds the jar. In certain cases, salt is added to the hot water sample, creating salty and humid vapor (in order to treat someone who reacts to the atmosphere in coastal climates). Samples of very hot water used in treatment of mild to moderate types of burns have shown excellent results. Cold, high altitude, low altitude, wind, dampness, dryness, rainwater, and other physical agents can be treated in a similar way.

Some patients react to heat or cold violently, suffering from extreme chills and shaking uncontrollably. They need to bundle up with three-four layers of clothing during a cold day or experience icy cold hands and feet even if they are clad in mittens and warm socks. These patients are simply allergic to cold and combinations with other substances. An allergy to cold makes the blood sticky and the circulation will be poor. The body will not be able to get rid of its toxins. Allergy to antioxidants like vitamin C, A, etc. makes the elimination of the toxins difficult. If patients are allergic to iron, hormones, heat, etc., their reactions are just the opposite in hot weather. They feel very uneasy in the heat. They may need treatments for vitamin C, iron, cold, hormones, and their own blood, alone or in combination. When they finish the treatment program, they are less prone to feeling cold or getting sick with the changes in temperature.

Genetic Factors

Discovery of possible tendencies toward allergies carried over from parents and grandparents opens a large door to achieving optimum health. Most people inherit the allergic tendency from their parents or grandparents. Allergies can also skip generations or manifest differently in parents from their children.

Bea, 38-years-old, had suffered from various allergies since she was an infant. When she was three-weeks-old, she broke out in a rash, which transformed into big heat boils. Her parents tried various medications in attempts to cure her; including allopathy, homeopathy, and herbal medicines. Finally, herbal medicine brought the problem somewhat under control. Even with the herbal treatment, she still occasionally suffered from outbreaks of skin lesions. When she was ten-years-old, she

*developed a type of severe migraine headaches, severe insomnia,
and mood swings, along with the arthritis.*

*After evaluation, she was found to be reacting to parasites.
We learned that both her parents were in the Peace Corps before
she was born. They were somehow infected with parasites and
were seriously ill for months, but had no idea that their health
problems were caused by the parasites until later. After she was
treated successfully with NAET for parasites, her health took a
quantum leap.*

Molds And Fungi

Molds and fungi are in a category by themselves because of
the numerous avenues through which they can come into contact
with people in everyday life. They can be ingested, inhaled,
touched, or even (as in the case of penicillin) injected. They can
also come in the form of airborne spores making up a large part of
the dust we breathe or pick up in our vacuum cleaners, in fluids
such as our drinking water, the dark fungal growth in the corners
of damp rooms. They can appear on the body as athlete's foot and
in particularly fetid vaginal conditions commonly called "yeast
infections." Molds and fungi also grow on trees and in the damp
soil, are a source of food (truffles and mushrooms), disease
(ringworm and the aforementioned yeast infections), and even of
medicine (penicillin).

Many children have severe allergy to sugar, starches, and
carbohydrates. Consumption and poor digestion of sugar products
cause to create yeast, candida, etc. in the gut of the person.
Overgrowth of these will cause them to travel to other parts of the
body. Molds and fungi, belong to the same family and share the
same energy fields. Reactions to these substances make children
irritable, depressed, and suffer from a variety of infections and
mental imbalances. When they get appropriate treatment to

eliminate their yeast, candida, mold and fungi, they become symptom-free.

Allergies to toilet papers, and baby wipes also cause yeast-like infections. Fungus and molds are found in the freezer too sometimes.

Emotional Factors

People suffer from various types of emotional allergies and blockages most of them caused by some form of allergies to what they eat, touch, breathe or come in contact with. When the allergens cause the blockages in the energy channels that supply to the brain, the brain will not receive proper nutrients to maintain the normal function. Just like the body, the brain also will begin to suffer from pain, discomfort and/or uneasiness. The pain, discomfort or uneasiness will manifest as headaches, asthma, migraines, blurred vision, dizziness, brain fog, shooting pains inside the brain, irritability, hyperactivity, autism, attention deficit disorders, learning disability, poor concentration, poor memory, crying spells, various exaggerated or abnormal sensations and feelings (e.g. fear, fright, disgust, anger, helplessness, frustration, low self-worth, obsession, hate, superiority or inferiority complexes, grief, etc.), phobias, unexplained pains anywhere in the body, indigestion, nausea, vomiting, anorexia, aversion to food, people, etc... the list of emotional symptoms arising from simple allergies can go on.

We need to recognize them, identify them, and eliminate them to achieve health in all three aspects --- ie. physical, physiological and emotional health. If one is free from energy blockages in these three levels, we can say that person is healthy.

From the time the world began, people from everywhere, all walks of life, all religions, all sects, all professions, have been searching desperately to find a way to achieve complete health in these three levels. Various medical practices gained some understanding and ways to manage the physical and physiological discomforts. People still do not understand the emotional aspect. When it came to the subject of emotional health, we lived in a kind of "dark age" until recently. No one gave any importance to emotional blockages and the diseases arising from them. For years people with emotional problems were treated badly. They were kept behind locked doors and/or in basements. Lay persons viewed mental illness as "possessions by demons," from which practice of "Exorcism" developed. Even now it is practised in various places by demon exterminators. The emotionally sick were tortured mistaking their emotional allergic reactions to some possessions. Later on when psychiatric medicine developed, they recognized the emotional imbalances but when these patients were sent to psychiatrists, they were labeled as "mentally ill," and institutionalized. Mental illness was completely perceived as a different disorder from a regular health disorder. No one made connection of emotional imbalances with food and environmental allergies, which could affect the emotional aspect of the meridian or organ. If the blockages remained at the emotional level for a long period of time, they can begin to affect physical and physiological levels in the body, eventually turning into a disease. Therefore, it is necessary to isolate and remove the cause of the emotional blockage as soon as possible. NAET deals with the whole body, removing blockages at the physical, physiological and emotional levels. Only then can a person be truly healthy.

Various emotional release techniques are being practiced in this country and in other countries. Some of them include: NAET Em Tech., Dianetics, La Chance Release method, Neuro-emotional technique, Thought field therapy (TFT), etc. Please find a practitioner near you and try to get some help if you think there is a problem in the emotional area.

Dear Dr. Devi,

I had to share this story with you. My little one has learned so much from you (so have I), here is how she handled a very emotional ongoing situation. Some relatives that she is close to and loves VERY much , sold their home and are moving out of the area. She has known this for some time now, but the full impact of their leaving just began. Because they are down sizing and do not have room, many of her special things including some of her pictures are now here at home in her room.

Last night I heard her sobbing. I went into her room and found her holding onto a picture of her with her aunt & uncle. I asked if I could do anything to help her and she asked that I stay close but not in her room. She actually cried and sobbed for almost 2 hours. This began about 10pm on a school night, I decided that I should respect her need to cry. I waited just down the hall. Then I heard her crying and talking out loud so I went to see what was going on. Dev was tapping her painful emotions on the emotional self-help points while talking out her sorrows just the way you have shown her. I left her alone and she continued to cry and talk and tap. At about 11:30pm she came out of her room to cuddle with me. I asked her how she was feeling and she responded in a giggle, " I tapped when I was crying the way Dr. Devi showed me, and I feel much better." Then she looked up and smiled and said " Thank you Mama, thank you Dr. Devi."

I know that she will still miss her favorite aunt and uncle, but the negative charge that was effecting her is gone.

Thank you Dr. Devi, so very much for loving us, all of us.

Barbara, Tarzana, CA

How about little infants and children? Do they have feelings? Do they have pain? Do they have emotions? No one really knows about that. No one seems to pay any attention to their feelings. How many of us really explain to the little ones about unusual events that take place around them in the household? Since they don't have the ability to communicate verbally, we assume that they don't know anything or they don't have any awareness of anything that takes place around them. If the parents or guardians would take time to introduce the family members and friends, explain to them of the unusual daily events (for example: fire in the house or neighborhood, earthquake, flood, death in the family, any new additions to the house, getting a new animal, wedding, etc.) they wouldn't have to grow up with so many emotional blockages. When they are brought from the hospital, we should make it routine to introduce all the family members to the infant. This may sound crazy to many but I have a feeling they understand everything as soon as they begin to see and hear. When they do not know who they are with, they get confused and scared and many children continue to grow up with that fear. I have treated many grown up patients with unknown fear leading to difficulty to live a normal life. Their problem clears up after treating for fears originated in infancy or childhood.

Fear From Infancy Was the Cause of His Asthma

Danny was suffering from asthma ever since he was an infant. His parents took him to the doctors and hospital emergencies very often. He was given inhalers and medications regularly. He suffered through his life with asthma until he was 25. He reacted to all animals. He loved to have a dog as a pet. But the sight of any animal triggered asthma in him. He came to see us for his asthma. He was found to be allergic to many food and environmental factors. After treating for all fifteen basics, he was treated for dried bean

mix. Dried bean mix had caused the energy blockage on his kidney meridians.

Fifteen minutes into his treatment, while still on the acupuncture therapy, he began an acute asthmatic attack. He had already failed the treatment for the dried bean mix. On further testing it was revealed that he was strong on the physical level and chemical level by muscle testing and weak on the emotional level. Further testing with NTT revealed that while he was six month old he was frightened by a black animal probably a dog, and that fear was the cause of his asthma. He had no awareness of such incident. His family had never mentioned anything like that before. So he was very surprised about this NTT discovery and eager to see the outcome of the treatment. I treated him with NAET-EM for the possible fear of that incident in infancy. In less than two minutes after the treatment, his wheezing stopped. Pink color spread through his face indicating that he was getting sufficient oxygen.

I advised him to call his mother to find out if there was in fact such an incident happened to him when he was six months old. I always took great interest in checking the validity of the NTT emotional findings. I have done that over and over for hundreds of times, but each case is a unique one and I insisted on doing that with each case and each incident. My friends often call me a "doubting Thomas," because of this nature. Danny went home and called his mother who lived in another city and shared with her all the happenings in my office. She couldn't remember anything immediately. But later in the evening she called him back saying the exciting news. Danny was lying on a mat in the living room floor while his mother was cooking in the kitchen and talking to her three cousins who were visiting them from New York. They heard sudden screaming cry from Danny and ran out to the sitting room. Their huge, black outdoor dog had somehow got inside and started sniffing the infant and the infant got frightened by the dog and began screaming out loud. They took the infant's inability to communicate verbally for granted and that infants do not have feelings. No one bothered to explain to the infant what had really happened there. If someone had the sense to explain to the child that everything is okay, this is just the family dog and he was just getting to know you by sniffing around, Danny may not have continued to be afraid of the animals until 25 years old. What else could have been a better action to protect everyone's interest? When the infant was brought from the hospital, someone should have introduced the infant to the dog properly (another family member who cannot talk?). Then dog wouldn't have had the anxiety and the excitement when it finally got a chance to meet the newcomer to the house. But how many of us pay attention to a dog's feelings when it comes to such matters?

Children could be having physical and chemical allergy towards his parents or vice versa. This could cause or lead to various health disorders. Parents should make a point to test the energy conflicts of the child between the mother, father, siblings, caretaker, baby sitter, friends, and their pets. If any energy difference is detected between the child and others involved with his/her care, it should be removed using NAET. NAET is the only method known so far that could treat person to person allergy or the allergy between human to human; human to animal; and animal to animal. Allergy between any of the above left untreated can cause a lot of discomfort in those involved and especially children.

My Granddaughter Was Allergic to Me!

Dear Dr. Devi,

My little granddaughter would not come near me. When I held out my arms to hold her, she would bury her head into the shoulder of whoever was holding her. If I had to take her to bathe or feed her, she would cry, get very cranky, aggressive, and irritable. At first I thought that she was tired, or teething. However, it happened constantly not to realize something was definitely amiss. I spoke to you and you immediately treated me for an allergy to my granddaughter. Two days later, when I saw my greatly loved grand baby—wonder of wonders—she ran into my arms! My first thought was to thank you, Dr. Devi.

My granddaughter continues to rush into my arms, her face lights up when she sees me, she smiles, laughs, and now plays a little game with me, which previously she had not done.

It's a miracle! I maintain my attitude of deepest gratitude to Dr. Devi, her expertise and her NAET treatment program.

Kindest Regards,
Marilyn D. Nordquist, Ph.D.
Rancho Palos Verdes, CA

She was allergic to her child!

When Lara was pregnant with Susanna, she suffered severe morning sickness. She was admitted in the hospital with hyperemesis graviderum on a couple of occasions due to excessive vomiting. She suffered from mild preeclampsia too. Finally when she delivered beautiful Susanna, she thought that was the end of her nine-months' misery. First two days in the hospital she felt great and slept very peacefully. Third day when she returned home, everything started all over. She began breast-feeding the infant. The infant refused to suck. Her breast got engorged and the pain was unbearable. Then she began having severe backache. 22 year old Lara had never known what a backache was before. For the first time in her life she knew what was backache. Her mother who was a hospital nurse said later, "her pain reaction resembled a kidney stone attack." She had seen them before. Her frightened family took her to the hospital. Had a complete examination and evaluation. There was no kidney stone. They couldn't find any cause for such intense pain. She was sent home with pain medication. In spite of the strong medication, she continued to be in pain. Four days later, she was brought to me recommended by one of the members from their church.

Testing with NTT, She was found to be not allergic to too many foods or environmental substances or chemical agents. She appeared to be a strongly built person. But further examination revealed that she was very allergic to her child physically and chemically and the child to her. I treated them for each other immediately using NAET and they had to avoid each other for 72 hours. Her mother took care of the infant for the next 72 hours since they showed the need to avoid each other for that long. A strong allergy indeed! Lara felt better instantly after the treatment. She continued to have mild backache for next 72 hours. When she came to the office she was supported by two people since she couldn't walk alone due to pain. When she left the office, she walked alone and with a smile. After 30 hours her backache reduced significantly, but it took 72 hour to pass the complete treatment. Lara never complained of her backache again and Susanna is a nine year old healthy girl now.

Many young children suffer from colic, insomnia, crying spells, temper tantrums, hyperactivity, restlessness, irritability, impatience, anger, behavioral problems, etc. The body may be projecting these symptoms hoping that someone would realize the presence of the adverse energy or energies in their energy field and help to remove them. When one cannot find any cause for the child's unusual behaviors, please use NTT and check for the presence of any adverse energies in their electromagnetic fields. You will be surprised to note how soon and with ease you could solve your child's puzzling problems.

CHAPTER 3

NAMBUDRIPAD'S TESTING TECHNIQUES

3

NAMBUDRIPAD'S TESTING TECHNIQUES

Symptoms of allergy vary from person to person depending upon the status of the immune system, age of the patient, severity of disease or degree of involvement of the organs and systems, and degree of inheritance. An allergy is a hereditary condition. An allergic predisposition is inherited, but may be manifested differently in family members.

There are many types of conventional allergy tests available to detect allergies; however, if it is done properly, the most reliable and convenient method of allergy testing is NTT testing. This is a modified form of kinesiological muscle testing. Allergies can be tested by NTT and treated very effectively with NAET. Please read Chapter 7 for more information on NTT and MRT.

Nambudripad's Testing Techniques

1. History

A complete history of the child is taken. A symptom survey form is given to the parents to record the level and type of discomfort the child is suffering.

2. Physical examination

Observation of the mental status, face, skin, eyes, color, posture, movements, gait, tongue, scars, wounds, marks, body secretions, etc.

3. Vital signs

Evaluation of pulse, skin temperature, and blood pressure, observation of swelling, growth, skin color, etc.

4. SRT

Skin Resistance Test for the presence or absence of a suspected allergen is done through a computerized electrodermal testing device if the child is four years or older; differences in the meter reading are observed (greater the difference from the base line reading, stronger the allergy).

The computerized tester also helps determine the various intensities of the allergies based on a 0 - 100 scale. This is probably one of the most accurate tests available today to determine allergies. The machine is designed to test food, environmental and chemical allergies, as well as allergies to molds, fungi, pollens, trees, grasses, proteins, vitamins, drugs, radiation, etc. It can be used to test allergies and their intensities before and after treatment so we are able to compare and show the body's response to the treatment.

The procedure does not involve breaking or puncturing the skin. There is no pain or discomfort. Hundreds of allergies can be tested on the patient in minutes. Since the testing probe only touches the skin for less than a second for each allergy tested, this method can be used for infants and children as well as adults. Another advantage of this machine is that it has a TV/computer monitor where the patient can read his/her own allergies as they are being recorded. A printout is produced and the data is saved for future comparison.

5. Blood Test For Eosinophils

Eosinophil count is usually seen high in children with food and environmental allergies.

6. Dynamometer Testing

Hand-held dynamometer can be used to measure and compare interphalangeal muscle strength (0-100) in the presence and absence of a suspected allergen. The dynamometer is held with thumb and index finger and squeezed to make the reading needle swing between 0-100 scale. Initial base line reading is observed first, then during contact with an allergen. The finger strength is compared in the presence of the allergen. If the second reading is more than the initial reading, there is no allergy. If the second reading is less than the initial reading, then there is an allergy. For example—if the initial (base line) reading is 40 on a scale of 1-100, and if the reading in the presence of an allergen (apple) is 28—the person is allergic to the apple. If the second reading is 60- or 70- there is no allergy. Another benefit of dynamometer testing is that the degree of the weakness/strength is measured in numbers. This gives us some understanding of the degree of allergy.

7. MRT To Detect Allergies

Muscle Response Testing is the body's communication pathway to the brain. Through MRT (testing through a surrogate), the child can be tested for various allergens. MRT is a standard test used in applied kinesiology to compare the strength of a predetermined test muscle in the presence and absence of a suspected allergen. If the particular muscle (test muscle) weakens in the presence of an item, it signifies that the item is an allergen. If the muscle remains strong, the substance is not an allergen. More explanation on MRT will be given in Chapter 7.

8. Amino Acid Analysis

Amino acid analysis can help you understand and treat a variety of health conditions such as chronic fatigue, food and chemical sensitivities, learning and behavioral disorders in children, and many neurological disorders.

9. ALCAT Test

One of today's most reliable and effective tests to detect allergies and sensitivities to food, chemicals, and food additives is the ALCAT test. This system is designed to measure blood cell reactions to foods, chemicals, drugs, molds, pesticides, bacteria, etc. The methodology of this simple test includes using innovative laboratory reagents allowing accurate cell measurement in their native form. Individually processed test samples, when compared with the "Master Control" graph, will show cellular reactivity (cell count and size) if it has occurred. Scores are generated by relating these effective volumetric changes in white blood cells to the control curve.

10. Scratch Test

Although other available methods of allergy testing are plentiful, traditional methods of testing have never been very reliable. Western medical allergists generally depend on skin testing, (scratch test, patch test, etc.), in which a very small amount of a suspected allergic substance is introduced into the person's skin through a scratch or an injection. The site of injection is observed for any reaction. If there is any reaction at that area of injection, the person is considered to be allergic to that substance. Each item has to be tested individually.

This manner of testing is more dangerous, painful and time-consuming than SRT. One has to be very careful when testing small children. Some patients can go into anaphylactic shock due to the introduction of extremely allergic items into the body. The painful procedure can cause soreness for several days. The patient must wait for a few days or weeks between tests because only one set of allergens can be tested at a time. This method is not very effective in identifying allergies to foods. Since it is not normal to inject foods under the skin, it is not surprising that there usually isn't a significant reaction.

11. Provocative/Neutralizing Technique

This test evaluates cellular immunity by determining patient response to the intradermal injection or topical application of one or more antigens. A minute amount of allergen (a weak dilution) is injected skin deep. It is strong enough to provoke the allergic symptoms in a person. The dilution and the amount of allergen used are noted. The allergen can produce skin erythema and/or wheal around the injected site. A record is kept of the amount, dilution and time injected. After a period of time, the size and shape of the wheal is observed. If the patient feels any reaction (dizzy spells, nausea, etc.), the tester will inject a smaller dose (weaker dilution) of the allergen that is capable of neutralizing the provocative action. This usually takes away the unpleasant symptoms or allergic reactions the patient felt from the initial injection. This is called the neutralizing dose. The neutralizing dose is used to relieve the allergic symptom and keep the patient under control for days.

12. Intradermal Test

The intradermal test is considered to be more accurate for food allergies than a plain scratch test. The name comes from the fact that a small portion of the extract of the allergen is injected intradermally, between the superficial layers of skin. Many people who show no reaction to the dermal or scratch type of testing show positive results when the same allergens are applied intradermally.

As in scratch tests, some patients can go into anaphylactic shock when extremely allergic items are injected into the body. The painful procedure can cause soreness for several days. The patient must wait a few days or weeks between tests, because only one set of allergens can be tested at a time.

13. Radioallergosorbant Test (RAST)

The radio-allergosorbant test or RAST measures IgE antibodies in serum by radioimmunoassay and identifies specific allergens causing allergic reactions. In this test, a sample of patient's serum is exposed to a panel of allergen particle complexes (APCs) on cellulose disks. Radiolabeled anti-IgE antibody is then added. This binds to the IgE-APC complexes. After centrifugation, the amount of radioactivity in the particular material is directly proportional to the amount of IgE antibodies present. Test results are compared with control values and represent the patient's reactivity to a specific allergen.

14. ELIZA

Another blood serum test for allergies is called the "ELIZA" (enzyme-linked immuno-zorbent assay) test. In this test, blood serum is tested for various immunoglobulin and their concentrations. Previous exposure to the allergen is necessary for this test to be positive in the case of an allergy. Eliza can identify an antibody or antigen, and replaces or supplements radioimmunoassay and immunofluorescence. To measure a specific antibody, an antigen is fixed to a solid phase medium, incubated with a serum sample. Then it is incubated with an anti-immunoglobulin-tagged enzyme. The excess unbound enzyme is washed from the system and a substrate is added. Hydrolysis of the substrate produces a color change, quantified by a spectrophotometer. The amount of antigen or antibody in the serum sample can then be measured. This method is safe, sensitive, and simple to perform and provides reproducible results. For this test to show some positive results the patient must be exposed to particular foods within a certain amount of time. If the patient has never been exposed to certain foods, the test results may be unsatisfactory.

15. EMF Test (Electro Magnetic Field Test)

The electromagnetic component of the human energy field can be detected with simple muscle response testing. The pool of electromagnetic energy around an object or a person allows the energy exchange. Human field absorbs the energy from the nearby object and processes through the network of nerve energy pathways. If the foreign energy field shares suitable charges with the human energy field, the human field absorbs the foreign energy for its advantage and becomes stronger. If the foreign energy field carries unsuitable charges, the human energy field causes repulsion from the foreign energy field. These types of reactions of the human field can be determined by testing an indicator muscle (specific muscle) before and during contact with an allergen. The electro- magnetic field of the humans or the human vibrations can also be measured by using the sophisticated electronic equipment developed by Dr. Valerie Hunt, Malibu, California. This genius researcher, a retired UCLA professor of physics, has proven her theory of the Science of Human Vibrations through 25 years of extensive research and clinical studies. Her book, "Infinite Mind" explains it all.

16. Sublingual Test

Another prevalent allergy test, which is used by clinical ecologists and some nutritionists, is called a sublingual test. It involves the instillation of a tiny amount of allergen extract under the tongue. If the test is positive, symptoms may appear very rapidly. The symptoms may include dramatic mental and behavioral reactions in addition to physical reactions. Some kinesiologists also use sublingual testing, but only for food items. A tiny amount of the food substance is placed under the tongue, and the patient is checked by muscle response testing.

17. Cytotoxic Testing

Cytotoxic testing is a form of blood test that was developed a few years ago. Many nutritionally oriented practitioners use this test. In this method, an extract of the allergic substance is mixed with a sample of the person's blood. It is then observed under the microscope for changes in white cells. Since foods and other allergic substances do not normally get into the blood in this manner, cytotoxic testing does not give reliable results.

18. Pulse Testing

Pulse testing is another simple way of determining food allergy. This test was developed by Arthur Coca M.D., in the 1950's. Research has shown that if you are allergic to something and you eat it, your pulse rate speeds up or slows down depending on the allergen's effect on sympathetic or parasympathetic nervous system. If it affects the sympathetic, pulse will speed up and para-sympathetic will slow it down.

Step 1:   Establish your base line pulse by counting radial pulse, or pedal pulse at the wrist for a full minute.

Step 2:   Put a small portion of the suspected allergen in a test tube and place it in the child's energy field (for example, place the test tube inside the socks, diaper, underpants, or under shirt, etc. for two minutes. Do not let the child eat the substance. The body contact with the substance will send the signal to the brain, which will send a signal through the sympathetic and parasympathetic nervous system to the rest of the body.

Step 3:   Retake the pulse with the allergen still in the energy field. An increase or decrease in pulse rate of 10% or more is considered an allergic reaction. The greater the degree of allergy the greater the difference in the pulse rate.

This test is useful to test food allergies, fabrics, chemicals, insects, etc. Make sure the allergen is inside the test tube with a lid. If your child is allergic to very many foods and if the child is consuming a few allergens at the same time, it will be hard to detect the exact allergen causing the reaction just by this test.

19. Blood Pressure Test

This test is similar to the pulse test. Systolic blood pressure reading is checked for changes in reading before and after the contact with the allergen.

Step 1:   Establish your base line by checking the systolic blood pressure.

Step 2:   Put a small portion of the suspected allergen in a test tube and place it in the child's energy field (for example, place the test tube inside the socks, diaper, underpants, or under shirt, etc. for two minutes. Do not let the child eat the substance. The body contact with the substance will send the signal to the brain, which will send a signal through the sympathetic and parasympathetic nervous system to the rest of the body.

Step 3:   Retake the systolic blood pressure with the allergen still in contact with the body. An increase in systolic blood pressure rate of 10% or more is considered an allergic reaction. The greater the degree of allergy the higher the blood pressure change will be.

20. The Elimination Diet

The elimination diet, which was developed by Dr. Albert H. Rowe of Oakland, California, consists of a very limited diet that must be followed for a period long enough to determine whether or not any of the foods included in it are responsible for the allergic symptoms. If a fruit allergy is suspected, for example, all fruits are eliminated from the diet for a specific period, which may vary from a few days to several weeks, depending on the severity of the symptoms. For patients who have suffered allergic symptoms over a period of several years, it is sometimes necessary to abstain from the offending foods for several weeks before the symptoms subside. Therefore, the importance of adhering strictly to the diet during the diagnostic period is very important. When the patient has been free of symptoms for a specific period, other foods are added, one at a time, until a normal diet is attained. This may not be very convenient for young children.

21. Rotation Diet

Another way to test for food allergy is through a "rotation diet," in which a different group of food is consumed every day for a week. In this method seven groups of food are consumed each week, with something different each day. The rotation starts again the following Monday. This way, reactions to any group can be traced and can be eliminated. All of these diets work better for people who are less reactive. The inherent danger in any of these methods is clear: If you are highly allergic to a certain food you can become very sick if you eat that item during testing even if you have not touched for years.

22. Like Cures Like

There are other allergy treatment methods in practice. Homeopaths believe that if an allergen is introduced to the patient in minute concentrations at various times, the patient can build up enough antibodies toward that particular antigen. Eventually, the patient's violent reactions to that particular substance may reduce in intensity. In some cases, reactions may subside completely and the patient can use or eat the item without any adverse reaction.

23. Sit With The Allergen In Your Palm

NAET patients are taught to test the allergen in another easy and safe way. Place a small portion of the suspected allergen in a baby food jar and ask the person to hold in her/his palm touching with the fingertips of the same hand for 15 minutes to 30 minutes. An allergic person will begin to feel uneasy when holding the allergen in his/her palm for a while giving rise to various unpleasant symptoms: begin to get hot, itching, hives, irregularities in heart beats (fast or slow heart beats), nausea, light headedness, etc. Since the allergen is inside the glass bottle, when such uncomfortable sensation is felt, the allergen can be put away immediately and hands washed to remove the energy of the allergen from the fingertips. This should stop the reactions immediately. In this way, the patient can detect out the allergens easily.

It is suggested that practitioner should have the patient tested for a couple of different diagnostic tests other than just MRT before and after completion of NAET. This can clearly document the progress of the patient and the effectiveness of NAET on each individual case.

All of the above methods work on a certain percentage of people. Curiously, people who had undergone all of these treatments were still found to be allergic to their identified allergies when they were tested again by muscle response testing. They still had to be treated by NAET to make them non-reactive.

CHAPTER 4

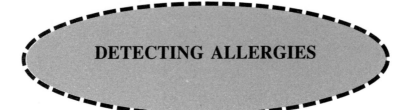

DETECTING ALLERGIES

4

DETECTING ALLERGIES

A detailed clinical history is the best diagnostic tool for any medical condition. It is extremely important for the patient or his/her parents or guardians to cooperate with the physician in giving all possible information about the child to the doctor in order to obtain the best results. It is my hope that this chapter will help bring about a clearer understanding between NAET specialists and their patients, because, in order to obtain the most satisfactory results, both parties must work together as a team.

The doctor should gather a detailed history of the child before formulating a diagnosis. Your doctor's office may ask you to complete a relevant questionnaire during your first appointment. It is important to cooperate with the office staff and provide as accurate a history as possible.

The Pediatric Patient-questionnaire

Prenatal history : socioeconomic factors, exposures to substance abuse, cadmium, lead, mercury, coffee, alcohol, chemical toxins, carbon monoxide poisoning, bacterial toxins, emotional traumas during fetal development, delivery, birth records including birth weight and APGAR scores.

Growth and Developmental History

Illnesses during early infancy?
- Colic——
- Constipation——
- Diarrhea——
- Feeding problem——
- Excessive Vomiting——
- Excessive white coating on the tongue ——
- Excessive crying ——
- Poor sleep ——
- Disturbed sleep ——
- Frequent ear infection ——
- Frequent fever ——
- Immunizations——
- Response to the immunizations ——
- Common childhood diseases like measles, chickenpox,
-       mumps, strep-throat, etc.——
- Any other unusual events (fire in the house, accidents, earthquakes, etc.)——

Developmental Milestones

Age of the child:
- Walked alone——
- Talked——
- Toilet trained for bladder and bowel——
- Enrolled in school——

Medical History

- Surgery—
- Hospitalizations——
- Diseases—
- Allergies—
- Frequent colds—
- Fevers—
- Ear infections—
- Asthma—
- Hives——
- Bronchitis—
- Pneumonia—
- Seizures—
- Sinusitis—
- Headaches—
- Vomiting —
- Diarrhea —
- Current medication—
- Any reaction to medication —
- Antibiotics and drugs taken —
- Parasitic infestation —
- Visited other countries —

Social History

Learning: grades at school, interaction between friends and teachers, interaction between family members, activities at school, phobias, and problems with discipline.

Behaviors: cooperative, uncooperative, disruptive and/or aggressive behaviors; overactive, restless, inattentive, day dreams; uncooperative with his/her peers and adults; incomplete or sloppy work.

Habits: temper tantrums, excessively active, constantly moving in seat or room, low self esteem, short attention span, poor memory, unusual fears, falls down often, clumsy, and unintentionally drops things.

Hobbies: reading, painting, singing, and riding, etc.

Family History

The medical history of the immediate relatives, mother, father, and siblings should be noted. The same questions are asked about the patient's distant relatives: grandparents, aunts, uncles, and cousins. A tendency to get sick or have allergies is not always inherited directly from the parents. It may skip generations or manifest in nieces or nephews rather than in direct descendants.

Commonly Asked Questions

Alcoholism, drug abuse, mental disorders, and other health disorders. The careful NAET specialist will also determine whether or not diseases such as tuberculosis, cancer, diabetes, rheumatic or glandular disorders exist, or have ever occurred in the patient's family history. All of these facts help give the NAET specialist a more complete picture of the hereditary characteristics of the patient. A *tendency* is inherited. It may be manifested differently in different people. Unlike the tendency, an actual medical condition such as diarrhea is not always inherited. Parents may have had cancer or rheumatism, but the child can manifest that allergic inheritance as Asthma.

Present History

When the family history is complete, the practitioner will need to look into the history of the patient's chief complaint and its progression. Some typical preliminary questions include: "When did your child's first symptom occur?" Did you notice your child's problem when he/she was an infant or a child, or did you first notice the symptoms during adolescence? Did it occur after going through a certain procedure? For example, did it occur for the first time after a dental procedure like applying braces or cleaning up a cavity? Did it happen the first antibiotic treatment or after installing a water filter? Did it occur after acquiring a water bed, a tricycle for instance or after a booster dose of immunization? One of my patients reported that her son's asthma began a few days after he received a pet (kitten) for his birthday.

Next, the doctor will want to know the circumstances surrounding and immediately preceding the first symptoms. Typical questions will include: "Did you change the child's diet or put him/her on a special diet? Did he/she eat something that he/she hadn't eaten lately, (perhaps for two or three months)? Did you feed him/her one type of food repeatedly, every day for a few days? Did the symptoms follow a childhood illness, (whooping cough, measles, chicken pox, diphtheria) or any immunization for such an illness? Did they follow some other illness such as influenza, pneumonia or a major operation? Did the problem begin after your vacation to an island, to another country, or after an insect bite? When did the first symptom appear?

Any one of these factors can be responsible for triggering a severe allergic manifestation or precipitate the first noticeable symptoms of an allergic condition. Therefore, it is very important to obtain full and accurate answers when taking the patient's medical history.

Other important questions relate to the frequency and occurrence of the attacks. Although foods may be a factor, if the symptoms occur only at specific times of the year, the trouble most likely is due to pollens. Often a patient is sensitive to certain foods but has a natural tolerance that prevents sickness until the pollen sensitivity adds sufficient allergens to throw the body into an imbalance. If symptoms occur only on specific days of the week, they are probably due to something contacted or eaten on that particular day.

The cause of disease can, at first, appear random. Regular attacks of rhinitis was caused in one patient after he worked on his coloring books. The colors caused a severe allergic reaction.

Another patient reacted similarly to the comic section of the newspaper. A boy always had a severe tension headache every day half way through his math class. He was allergic to the math book. Another boy had migraines on the days he went to school. He was accused of being lazy and parents and teachers punished him for not wanting to go to school. The cause was traced to eating a kind of cereal before he went to school. He did not eat the cereal on his days off. After he was treated for that particular cereal, he did not get his migraines anymore. Another child had an allergic attack of sneezing, runny nose, mental irritability, and headaches on Saturdays. I traced the allergy to the shampoo her mother used to wash her hair with on Friday afternoons.

The time of day when the attacks occur is also of importance in determining the cause of an allergic manifestation. If it always occurs before mealtime hypoglycemia may be a possible cause. If it occurs after meals, an allergy to carbohydrates and starch complexes or something in the meal should be suspected. If it occurred regularly at night, it is quite likely that there is something in the bedroom that is aggravating the condition. It may be that the patient is sensitive to: feathers in the pillow or comforter, wood cabinets, marble floors, carpets, side tables, end tables, bed sheets, pillows, pillow cases, detergents used in washing clothes, indoor plants, shrubs, trees, or grasses outside the patient's window.

One of my patients suffered from severe insomnia and irritability at night. After spending a few minutes in bed, he regularly got up agitated and uptight and spent the rest of the night without sleep. He was found to be allergic to his blue colored silk bed sheet and pillow cases; he was found to be allergic to the color blue, which instead of calming him, made him agitated and irritable.

Many patients react violently to house dust, different types of furniture, polishes, house plants, tap water and purified water. Most of the city water suppliers change the water chemicals only once or twice a year. Although, this is done with good intentions, people with chemical allergies may get sicker if they ingest the same chemicals over and over for months or years. Contrary to traditional western thinking, developing immunity can be the exception rather than the rule.

Occasionally, switching the chemicals around gives allergic patients a change of allergens and a chance for them to recover from the existing reactions. In this way, repeated use of the same chemicals can be avoided.

Across the United States, chlorination is used as the primary disinfectant in water systems. Although chlorination will kill most of the bacteria, viruses are not destroyed by any of these cleansing processes. Tri-halomethanes, which are a by-product of chlorine, are also used to clean the water. Ozone is used as a disinfectant for drinking water. Some of these chemicals are known to cause birth defects, nervous system disorders, damage to body organs and many other irreversible sicknesses.

The doctor should ask the patient to make a daily log of all the foods he/she is eating. The ingredients in the food should be checked for possible allergens. Certain common allergens like corn products, MSG (monosodium glutamate or Accent), citric acid, etc. are used in food preparations.

Allergy to corn is one of today's most common allergies, especially in young children. Unfortunately, cornstarch is found in almost every processed food and some toiletries and drugs too. Chinese food, baking soda, baking powder, and toothpaste contain large amounts of cornstarch. It is the binding product in almost all vitamins and pills, including aspirin and Tylenol. Corn syrup is the natural sweetener in many of the products we ingest, including soft drinks. Corn silk is found in cosmetics and corn oil is used as a vegetable oil. For sensitive people this food adds another nightmare.

Other common ingredients in many preparations that children may react severely to are the various gums (acacia gum, xanthine gum, karaya gum, etc.). Numerous gums are used in candy bars, yogurt, cream cheese, soft drinks, soy sauce, barbecue sauce, fast food products, macaroni and cheese, etc.

Carob, a staple in many health food products, is another item that causes brain irritability among allergic people. Many health-conscious people are turning to natural food products in which carob is used as a chocolate and cocoa substitute. It is also used as a natural coloring or stiffening agent in soft drinks, cheeses, sauces, etc. We discovered that some of the causes of "holiday flu" and suicide attempts are allergies to carob, chocolate, and turkey.

If your child has allergies you must look for these ingredients and additives in the food products you buy from the market.
Please read the labels. Manufacturers usually list these items on the cover of the product-container.

Acetic Acid (sodium acetate and sodium diacetate). This is a common food additive. This is the acid of vinegar. Acetic acid is used as an acidic flavoring agent for pickles, sauces, catsups, mayonnaise, wine, foods that are preserved in vinegar, some soft drinks, processed cheese, baked goods, cheese spreads, sweet and sour drinks and soups. It is also naturally found in apples, cocoa, coffee, wine, cheese, grapes, and other over-ripened fruits. If your child gets allergic reaction to these natural foods he/she may be allergic to acetic acid.

Agar (Seaweed extract): This is a polysaccharide that comes from several varieties of algae and it can turn like a gel if you dissolve it in water. So this is used in ice cream, jellies, preserves, icings, laxatives, used as a thickening agent in milk, cream, and used as gelatin (vegetable form). This is a safe additive, but if your child is allergic to sea foods you may need to eliminate the allergy for this.

Albumin (cow milk-albumin): Many children are allergic to albumin in the milk. Researchers have found children/people who are allergic to milk albumin are at high risk to get any of these disorders: ADD, ADHD, Autism, bipolar diseases, schizophrenia, and other allergy-related brain disorders. NAET can desensitize you for milk-albumin.

Aldicarb: It is an organic chemical water pollutant, seen often in city water. When the concentration of this chemical gets high in the city water, many people get sick with gastrointestinal disorders, like nausea, vomiting, pain, bloating, stomach flu, etc. Boiling the water for 30 minutes could help reduce the reaction. If your child is not allergic to apple cider vinegar, adding two-three drops of vinegar in eight ounces of water might help.

Alginates (Alginic acid, algin gum, ammonium, calcium, potassium, and sodium alginates, propylene glycol alginates): Most of these are natural extracts of seaweed and used in the food industry primarily as stabilizing agents.

Propylene glycol is an antifreeze. This is supposed to be a safe solvent, used in food preparation, especially in ice creams. Alginates help to retain water. It helps to prevent ice crystal formation; helps uniform distribution of flavors through foods. They add smoothness and texture to the products and are used in ice creams, custards, chocolates, chocolate milk, cheese, salad dressings, jellies, confections, cakes, icings, jams, and some beverages.

Aluminum Salts (alum hydroxide, alum potassium sulfate, sodium alum phosphate, alum ammonium sulfate, and alum calcium silicate).: Aluminum salts are used as a buffer in various products. This helps to balance the acidity. Used as an astringent to keep canned produce firm, to lighten food texture, and used as an anti-caking agent.

Sodium aluminum phosphate is used in baking powder and in self-rising flours. Alum is used as a clarifier for sugar and as a hardening agent. Aluminum hydroxide is used as a leavening agent in baked goods. It is a strong alkali agent that can be toxic but when used in small amounts it is fairly safe. It is also used in antiperspirants and antacids. Aluminum ammonium sulfate is used as an astringent, and neutralizing agent in baking powder and cereals. It can cause burning sensation to the mucous membranes. Overuse of aluminum products may lead to aluminum toxicity and it can affect the brain chemistry. Other sources of aluminum are cookware, deodorants, antacids, aluminum foils, cans and containers.

Benzoates (sodium benzoate).: Benzoic acid occurs naturally in anise, berries, black olive, blueberries, broccoli, cauliflower, cherry bark, cinnamon, cloves, cranberries, ginger, green grapes, green peas, licorice, plums, prunes, spinach, and tea. Benzoic acid or sodium benzoate is commonly used as a preservative in food processing. This is used as a flavoring agent in chocolate, orange, lemon, nut, and other flavors in beverages, baked products, candies, ice creams, and chewing gums and also used as a preservative in soft drinks, margarine, jellies, juices, pickles, and condiments.

This is also used in perfumes and cosmetics to prevent spoilage by microorganisms. Benzoic acid is a mild antifungal agent. It is metabolized by the liver. Large amount of benzoic acid or benzoates can cause intestinal disturbances, can irritate the eyes, skin, and mucous membranes. This causes eczema, acne and other skin conditions in sensitive people.

Cal. Proprionate: (sodium proprionate and proprionic acid): These are found in dairy products, cheese, breads, cakes, baked goods and chocolate products, They are used as preservatives and mold inhibitors. They reduce the growth of molds and some bacteria.

Source: Baked products, breads, rolls, cakes, cup cakes, processed cheese, chocolate products, preserves, jellies, and butter.

Cal. Silicate: Used as an anticaking agent in products, table salt and other foods preserved in powder form used as a moisture control agent.

Carbamates: These pesticides are used widely in many places. Their toxicity is slightly lesser than some other pesticides like organochlorines. They are known to produce birth defects.

Source: pesticide-sprayed foods.

Carbon Monoxide: CO is an odorless, colorless gas that competes with oxygen for hemoglobin. The affinity of CO for hemoglobin is more than 200-fold greater than that of oxygen. CO causes tissue hypoxia. Headache is one of the first symptoms, followed by confusion, decreased visual acuity, tachycardia, syncope, metabolic acidosis, retinal hemorrhage, coma, convulsions, and death.

Source: Driving through heavy traffic, damaged gas range, leaky valves of the gas line, exhaust pipes, living in a closed up room for long time, trapped firewood smoke, smoke inhalation from being in a closed, running car, an automobile kept running in closed garage for hours, exhaust from autos and other machinery, etc.

Casein: Milk protein. Also used in prepared foods, candies, protein shakes, etc.

EDTA: This is a very efficient polydentate chelator of many divalent or trivalent cations including calcium. This is used primarily in lead poisoning. This is toxic to the kidneys. Adequate hydration is necessary when you take this in any form.

Ethylene gas (used on fruits, especially on green bananas).

Food Bleach: Most of these are used in bleaching the flour products. Benzoil peroxides, chlorine dioxides, nitrosyl chlorides, potassium bromate, mineral salts, potassium iodate, ammonium sulfate, ammonium phosphate, are the most commonly used food bleaches. They whiten the flour. They also improve the appearance. Whatever they are using should be listed on the labels. Sometimes more than one item is used for better benefit.

Formic Acid: This is a caustic, colorless, forming liquid. Naturally seen in ants (ant bite), synthetically produced and used in tanning and dyeing solutions, fumigants and insecticides. This is also used as an artificial flavoring in food preparations.

Malic Acid: A colorless, highly water soluble, crystalline substance, having a pleasant sour taste, and found in apples, grapes, rhubarb, and cactus. This substance is found to be very effective in reducing general body aches. If you are allergic to it, then you can get severe body ache.

Mannan: Polysaccharides of mannose, found in various legumes and in nuts. Allergy to this factor in dried beans causes fibromyalgia-like symptoms in sensitive people.

Mannitol: It is hexahydric alcohol, used in renal function testing to measure glomerular filtration. Used intravenously as an osmotic diuretic.

Salicylic Acid: Amyl, phenyl, benzyl, and methyl salicylates).

A number of foods including almonds, apples, apricots, berries, plums, cloves, cucumbers, prunes, raisins, tomatoes, and wintergreen. Salicylic acid made synthetically by heating phenol with carbon dioxide is the basis of acetyl salicylic acid. Salicylates are also used in a variety of flavorings such as strawberry, root beer, spice, sarsaparilla, walnut, grapes, and mint.

Succinic Acid: Found in meats, cheese, fungi, and many vegetables with its distinct tart, acid taste.
Source: asparagus, broccoli, beets, and rhubarb.

Talc (magnesium silicate): Talc is a silica chalk that is used in coating, polishing rice and as an anticaking agent. It is used externally on the body surface to dry the area. Talc is thought to be carcinogenic. It may contain asbestos particles. White rice is polished and coated with it.

Tartaric Acid: This is a flavor enhancer. It is a stabilizer.

Commonly seen Water Chemicals (in drinking water).
Alum sulfate, ammonium chloride, benzene, carbon tetrachloride, chlorine, DDT, ferric chloride, gasoline, heavy metals (mercury, silver, zinc, arsenic, lead, copper), organochlorides, organophosphates, PCBs, pesticides, petroleum products, Sodium hydroxide, toluene, and xylene.

Commonly seen Water pollutants: There are many water pollutants we see in our water. Some of them get filtered out by the time we receive in our tap. Most of these pollutants still remain in small amounts. Some of these are inorganic water pollutants like: arsenic, asbestos, cadmium, chromium, copper, cyanide, Lead, mercury, nickels, nitrates, nitrosamines, selenium, silica, silver, and zinc.

Organic chemical water pollutants: 1,2, dichloroethane, 2,4,5,T, 2,4,-D., aldicarb, benzene, carbon tetrachloride, chloroform, DDT, dioxane, dibromo-chloropropane (DBCP), dichlorobenzene, ethylene dibromide (EDB), gasoline, lindane, polychlorinated biphenyls (PCB), polynuclear aromatic hydrocarbon (PAH), tetrachloroethylene, toluene, toxaphene, trichloromethane, trichloroethylene (TCE), vinyl chloride, MTBE (Methyl tertiary butyl ether is a gasoline additive), and xylene.

Some people with extreme sensitivity to these pollutants react badly with exposure by exhibiting mild to severe symptoms in various health areas. Some of the commonly seen symptoms are nausea, vomiting, diarrhea, abdominal cramps, brain fog, fatigue, body ache, joint pains, water retention in the body, flu like symptoms, fever, eczema, and rashes, sinusitis, post nasal drips, insomnia, etc. If you boil it for 30 minutes, the effect of these chemicals is reduced.

When assessing a child, care must be taken not to misdiagnose him/her. Misdiagnosis can hurt the child and his/her family's peace of mind for a long time.

As I have stated earlier, in my opinion, the children who get labelled with various childhood disorders may be suffering from simple undiagnosed allergies. Many food and environmental allergic symptoms overlap or mimic a variety of diseases including many neurological and brain disorders.

After completing the patient's history, the NAET specialist should examine the patient for the usual vital signs. A physical examination is performed to check for any abnormal growth or condition. If the patient has an area of discomfort in the body, it should be inspected. It is important to note the type and area of discomfort and its relationship to an acupuncture point. Most pain and discomfort in the body usually occurs around some important acupuncture point.

Twelve meridians combined with their channels and branches cover almost every part of the human body. The NAET specialist should examine all these meridians and branches for possible energy blockages. An acupuncturist is trained to understand the exact location of the pathways of these meridians. For this reason, the exact symptoms are very important. By identifying the symptoms, you can identify the area of the energy blockage. From this location, the experienced acupuncturist/ NAET specialist can detect the meridians, organs, muscles and nerve roots associated with the blockage. The NAET specialist will then be able to make an appropriate diagnosis by evaluating the presenting symptoms (read Chapter 7 for possible pathological symptoms) and determine what particular allergen is causing the specific problem. When the source of the problem is identified, treatment becomes easier.

CHAPTER 5

PEDIATRIC ALLERGIES PART-1

5

PEDIATRIC ALLERGIES
PART-1

Statistics indicate that approximately 3–5% of school-age children in the United States have been diagnosed as suffering from some form of allergy and related diseases. My experience has shown that most of the cases of childhood illnesses are the result of undiagnosed allergies.

The shocking fact is that there are hardly any human diseases or conditions in which allergic factors are not involved directly or indirectly. Any substance under the sun, including sunlight itself, can cause an allergic reaction in any individual. In other words, potentially, you can be allergic to anything you come in contact with and these allergies can make you sick or at least put you "under the weather." If you learn how to test and find your allergies, in other words if you can learn how to find the cause of your illness before it produces an illness in you or in your child, you and your child could avoid the illnesses and do not have to get sick at all. Now you have a way to do just that. You can test and find your allergies within the privacy of your own home, without going through expensive and extensive laboratory tests. Using the simple NAET self-help procedures described in Chapter 9, and utilizing the simple home remedies given after each health condition, you may be able to help your child's most frequently seen, common health problems within your own home. After trying these simple self-help remedies if your child continues to express symptoms without showing any improvement, please consult an NAET specialist for further guidance, evaluation and treatments. If you take time to read this book, it is easy to learn to evaluate your child's simple health problems. For complicated problems, you need to consult the appropriate specialists.

We are living in a scientifically and technologically advanced world where the vendors and merchants are in great competition to bring out their new products to each and everyone. Each and every product stands out for it's own quality and the consumers give in to their temptation by using them. The new products are also filling up our environment (pesticides, insecticides, cleaning agents, chemical sprays, chemical purifiers in the city water and other bottled drinking water, plastics and vinyl products, different kinds of fabrics, colors, fabrics treated with different kinds of chemicals, various types of radiation from television, laser equipments, cellular phones, etc., to name a few). Science and technology have altered the life-style of mankind enormously. The reactions and diseases arising from responses to these changes are also very different. These new inventions have changed the quality of our lives dramatically and without these technological inventions, we would be still living in dark ages. I don't think anyone would want to return to the old times where no one used pesticides and didn't suffer from seizure disorders and multiple sclerosis or malaria, but died from bug poison or parasite infestation. In the old days, no one used chemical cleaning agents and didn't suffer from breathing disorders and eczema, but died from bacterial infections. Our chemical explosion and advanced technology have found an end to the health disorders brought on by pests and bugs in many people and improved the life-styles of many people dramatically. Yet, these same inventions and scientific accomplishments have become everlasting nightmares for some people and their children who are allergy prone.

Technology is becoming more pervasive over time. Let's face it, technology will always be with us. It is hard to change and no one who has seen the changes in civilization and its benefits would want to go back to old times. We cannot deny the magical benefits of telephones, automobiles, airplanes, computers, internet and web sites to name a few. But allergic patients must find ways to overcome adverse reactions to new chemicals and other allergens created by the new technology they are exposed to. This is not good news to the sensitive people. The new products are generating new types of allergies causing new types of illnesses. Hospitals are filled with emergencies; doctors' clinics are overflowing and understaffed to handle the number of desperate patients showing up in their offices every day. Another problem adding to this dilemma is that no one really knows the exact cause of the patients' problems. A scapegoat diagnosis is issued for all these new modern-day problems. The plan of treatment is focused on symptom-oriented or symptomatic treatments.

When someone comes to a doctor's office with a common cold, flu, runny nose, sinus congestion, sinusitis, brain fog, asthma, stomach ache, backache, headache, migraine, body ache, pain in the leg, restless leg syndrome, not feeling like going to school, not feeling like studying, not feeling like talking to anyone one day, how many of the doctors take time to find a cause to these problems before prescribing a medication or a symptomatic treatment? We learn in medical schools to treat the symptoms of a patient and make the patient symptom-free and happy. Our usual practice is that we don't really look into the cause unless it is a complicated problem. When the symptom relieves temporarily, patients and doctors are happy but they forget that the next attack awaits in the corner as long as the cause is unknown.

NAET will fit right in with the 21st century life-style of the modern world. Even though it requires a series of detailed treatments, NTT and NAET, (Nambudripad's Allergy Elimination treatments) offer the prospect of relief to adults and their children who suffer from constant provocations from modern-day allergies.

NAET is slightly different from the usual existing medical practice. It is designed to be a cause-oriented treatment plan. NAET teaches you to find out the root cause of a problem, then eliminate it, so that the symptoms may not return. Simple problems of your life can be taken care of using simple methods, so that everyone with a problem small or big do not have to go to hospitals or to a busy doctor's offices. Real needy patients can go to the hospitals and/or to the doctors' offices. This will help the hospitals to function efficiently providing best care to the needy patients preventing unnecessary hospital admissions to people with simple problems. This will also prevent the overcrowding of the doctors' offices. How can the patient or parents benefit from this? You will have enough quality time to spend with your healthy child and use the money that you would spend on unnecessary medical care wisely and productively.

You will change your perception about diseases dramatically after you learn about NAET. For example: when someone gets a common cold (nasal blockages or runny nose, sore throat, sneezing, feeling chills, etc.), you may immediately look for a new or different item you ate, drank, touched or inhaled within the last few hours. You may write down every item that you came in contact with and test each item using NAET-MRT to find out which item made your MRT weak. When you isolate the weak item (for example the orange juice you drank at breakfast), immediately you may treat that item using NAET. To your amazement, you may find that a few minutes after the NAET treatment for the orange juice, you do not suffer from any more cold symptoms. NAET can produce such magical on-the-spot results if learned and practiced correctly.

To achieve this kind of testing and treating ability one needs to learn to test properly by MRT. This comes only by practice... hours of dedicated practice.

Some might say "it is not easy to learn NTT or NAET -- - testing is difficult --- can't get accurate results by MRT, etc." In fact MRT is the most accurate testing I have found so far. MRT is easy to do. You need to work hard initially to learn it and master it just like anything else. You will be amazed at your own test results once you learn it. Read this book as many times as you need if you are not familiar with acupuncture, chiropractic, kinesiology, energy medicine, etc. You need to find a partner and read and practice the techniques in Chapter 7 to master the testing skill. You need to spend more time on these chapters (Chapters 5&6) and the next one if you would like to look for commonly seen allergens in relation to most often seen childhood health disorders.

As stated earlier you can be allergic to: foods, drinks, drugs, childhood immunizations, herbs, vitamins, city water, drinking water, clothing, jewelry, cold, heat, wind, food colors, additives, preservatives, chemicals, formaldehyde, etc. Undiagnosed allergies can produce symptoms of various health disorders including the common ailments we see in our children.

By learning the simple Nambudripad's Testing Technique (NTT in Chapter 7), anyone can easily learn to recognize various allergens and the health problems they cause. This will help the sufferer begin to seek the appropriate diagnostic studies and pursue proper health care as needed without wasting time. When the patient's diagnosis is correct, results are less frightening.

An allergic reaction may be manifested in varying degrees as mild to severe irritability of any organ system causing itching, rashes, hives, edema, asthma, joint pains, muscle aches, headaches, restlessness, insomnia, addictions, craving, indigestion, vomiting, anger, depression, irritability, hyperactivity, disturbed vision, poor attention span, panic attacks, brain fatigue, and brain fog. This clearly points out that there are no typical responses to allergens in the real world. If we are depending on allergies to produce a uniform set of responses for all people, we may misdiagnose and provide the wrong treatment. We cannot duplicate and package a standard medication as an antidote for any specific allergy—each individual case is different. We must not oversimplify our treatment of patients. Not everyone exhibits typical allergic symptoms (whatever we perceive typical to be). Should we do so, we risk missing a myriad of potential reactions that may be produced in some people in response to their contact with substances that are for them allergens.

You may continue all other medications you are using on your child while you follow the treatments. There are no contraindication with NAET if you want to give any other treatments or products while the child is receiving NAET. Please check the allergy to the drugs, vitamins, skin creams, etc. before using them on the child.

We cannot ignore the scientific achievements of the drug industry. Sometimes drugs are useful or necessary to control the acute symptoms. Lately, powerful herbs and vitamins are replacing some drugs. There is nothing wrong in using drugs or vitamins to reduce or control the severe symptoms when it is needed. If they don't agree with your system, drugs and vitamins cannot do the expected job. They both can damage your system. How can you get the best out of drugs or vitamins?

There are certain rules for the successful usage of drugs or supplements.

• First, and most importantly, the practitioner should check the drug and supplements for any possible allergy.

• Drugs should be used wisely and only when it is absolutely necessary.

• Drugs should be used only to achieve a short term goal.

• The cause of the problems should be identified and eliminated as soon as possible.

The drug should be replaced with a nonallergic, natural effective substitute (therapy, herbs etc.) soon after the acute problem is solved.

Sometimes, drug usage is necessary even in the treatments with NAET. I encourage the use of drugs in the initial stages of NAET treatments when it is necessary. If the presenting symptoms are kept under control, NAET treatments will work better. But one problem I often encounter is that most people are reactive and highly allergic to the very drug that is supposed to help them stabilize their body functions. In such situation if one uses drugs they can harm the child more than the disease itself. Doctors who prescribe drugs should learn to test the possibility of getting an allergic reaction to the drug and/or supplements before they are prescribed to the little children. The parents also should learn the simple NTT testing procedures so that they can help their children from unexpected and unpleasant reactions from drugs or supplements.

Children suffer from various side effects of drugs and supplements: immunizations, vaccinations, and vitamin supplements (concentrated vitamins are dangerous if the child is allergic to them). The reactions vary greatly in manifestations and intensity. Some of the commonly seen reactions are: mild skin rashes to severe hives all over the body, indigestion to severe vomiting and diarrhea, tiredness to extreme fatigue, shortness of breath to severe asthma, and fainting to anaphylaxis. So before prescribing any drug, the practitioner should test the patient carefully for a possible allergy to the drug before prescribing it. If found, it should be treated immediately. An allergy to drugs can harm the patient more than any other toxin you can think of. Allergy and its side effects can easily be tested using NTT. After successful elimination of the allergen, the patient will be able to use it as needed to keep his/her other symptoms under control.

Every child should be tested and treated for all NAET group-A, these are the basic treatments. NAET basic treatments include the most commonly used food and environmental substances in every day life. If a child is allergic to all the essential nutrients, he can become reactive to everything else around him/her. By eliminating the allergies to the essential nutrients, child's immunity will improve or maintain at a very high level with the result that your child may not get other allergies or allergy based illnesses as often as the other children who have not had NAET treatments. This will give him/her the chance to grow healthy, happy and productive in school and later at work, without having to fight allergies and illnesses.

NAET basic allergen groups: there are 50 major groups. Most preferred order of treatments is given in Classic NAET group - 80% of the allergic reactions will diminish if one clears on all these allergens. According to the symptoms these allergen groups can be rearranged or after the basic thirteen, allergens can be treated by the necessity of the child's immediate problem. It is called "treatment by priority."

Classic NAET Group

1. Egg mix
2. Calcium mix
3. Vitamin C mix
4. B complex
5. Sugar mix
6. Iron mix
7. Vitamin A mix
8. Minerals
9. Salt Mix
10. Grains
11. Yeast mix, yogurt and whey
12. Artificial sweeteners
13. Coffee, Chocolate and caffeine
14. Spice mix 1 & 2
15. Vegetable fat & animal fat
16. Nut mix-1 & Nut mix-2
17. Fish and Shell fish
18. Amino Acids 1 & 2
19. Whiten-all
20. Turkey/Serotonin
21. Fluoride
22. Gum mix
23. Dried Bean mix
24. Alcohol
25. Gelatin
26. Vegetable mix
27. Vitamin D
28. Vitamin E
29. Vitamin F (fatty acids)
30. Vitamin T (Thymus gland)
31. RN.A. & D.N.A.
32. Stomach acids
33. Base (Digestive enzymes)
34. Food Coloring
35. Food Additives
36. Starch mix
37. Nightshade vegetables
38. Virus mix
39. Bacteria Mix
40. Parasites
41. Chemicals
42. Pollens
43. Grasses/weeds
44. Formaldehyde
45. Latex/plastics
46. Crude oil/Synthetic materials
47. Animal epithelial/dander
48. Smoking/Nicotine
49. Dust/ Dust mites
50. Perfume mix/ Flowers

NAET GROUP-A

1. Egg mix
2. Calcium mix
3. Vitamin C mix
4. B complex
5. Sugar mix
6. Iron mix
7. Vitamin A mix
8. Minerals
9. Salt Mix
10. Grains / corn mix
11. Yeast mix, yogurt and whey
12. Stomach Acid.
13. Base / Digestive enzymes

Some of the commonly seen pediatric allergies and childhood disorders arising from such pediatric allergies are given below. NAET testing procedures (also called NTT) are given in Chapter 7. NAET self-help for some of these conditions are given following each condition and also described in Chapter 9 of this book. Please read it carefully and understand it before you apply on a child. The self-help section does not replace the need for a health practitioner. It may give you some quick relief until you can get to your doctor. You should consult your NAET doctor for eliminating the allergies as soon as the acute problem is taken care of so that you could most often prevent future encounters of the similar problems.

Using NTT testing procedures find the causative agent if possible and avoid the allergen. If you cannot test properly find the nearest NAET practitioner for help. You can get the NAET practitioner's names from NAET practitioner locator section from our site **"www.naet.com"** Your practitioner will try to eliminate the allergy to the immediate causative agent if it is an acute problem. If it is a chronic problem, he/she will treat the NAET basic ten-fifteen and then treat the specific allergen. NAET treatments can give quicker and lasting relief if done properly.

During the initial stages of treatments, we like you to support your system with nonallergic, healing herbs, vitamins and minerals. Some of the suggested home remedies are easily found in your kitchen shelf. Some of you may already know these remedies. The suggested special vitamins and Chinese herbs are available from your NAET practitioner to help with your symptoms temporarily and promote healing. These herbal supports sholud be used only as needed. You should stop them as soon as the symptoms get contolled. Suggested dose is for children between 2-10 years of age. Reduce it to half for infants and toddlers until two or increase the dosage for bigger children. The NAET supplementation protocol given in Chapter 9 may help you to adjust the dosage for your child. Do not self medicate. Herbs can be dangerous if taken inappropriately. Check with your doctor before you take it or give it to your child. Check the resource section in the back of this book for the addresses of the vitamins and herb companies. If you are not a health professional you may not be able to order them directly.

Acupressure help points are given after each condition. Massaging these points gently clockwise for 1-3 minutes can give temporary relief.

Before giving any of the suggested teas, vitamins, herbs, mineral supplements, items used for inhalations, sitz baths, local applications and other therapeutic products should be checked for any possible allergy using MRT and if found the allergy should be eliminated before using the product or procedure. If it is difficult to treat or unable to treat, please do not use the product. (Read Chapters 7 and 9 for instructions in order to test and evaluate the allergens. In addition, you can also find guidance for preparation of special teas, drinks, baths, soaks, and NAET supplementation procedures and how to find your child's correct dosage of the medication, vitamin, and other supplements in Chapter 9. Please read and understand the procedure before you work with your child).

Infectious Mononucleosis

This is one of the commonly seen childhood disorders. This is caused by Epstein-Barr virus, characterized by fever, pharyngitis, and swelling of the lymph nodes. Fatigue is common in the first two-three weeks. Fever usually peaks in the afternoon or early evening with temperatures between 103-105 degrees.

NAET HELP

Find the causative agent if possible and treat with NAET child-help protocol (Read Chapters 7 and 9 for instructions).

Collect a sample of the child's saliva at the first sign of the disease and treat daily with NAET until the symptoms are under control; if the disease has already progressed, then treat also a sample of urine, body secretion, sweat, or stool three times a day for a week using child-help protocol.

Treat for classic NAET group with a practitioner.

ACUHELP: Massage SP-10 four times a day for 1 minute each time. Add LI-11 along with SP-10 if the child has fever.

Supplements

(Suggested doses are for children between age 2-10 years. Some of the names of the herbal companies are given in the resource section of this book. Only a licensed medical practitioner can order the products from these companies).

Garlic 1 clove or kayolic 1 pill (100 mgs) twice a day.

Coriander (cilantro seed or leaves) tea 1 ounce twice a day.

Astragalus herb 1 gram daily.

Immuplex 1 three times daily for 6 weeks.

Calcium lactate, vitamin C with bioflavinoids, vitamin B complex, vitamin A, and trace minerals as needed after clearing for allergies. (Check the dosage using NAET -supplement test).

Fever of Unknown Origin

If a child has a rectal fever of 103 degrees taken on four different occasions over a two-week period with no apparent cause, he/she is said to be having a *fever of unknown origin*. Some types of allergy may be the origin. The allergic reaction can turn into an inflammation of the affected tissue. Inflammation attracts virus and bacteria. So an infection follows an inflammation. Infection accounts for about 50% of the fevers of unknown origin. Almost 50% of these are due to viruses and 65% are in children <2 years old. Children tend to attract virus and bacteria more than grown up people. Nonspecific symptoms (fatigue, chills, and sweats) are common. In our society, at some point in the illness 80% of the children receive antibiotics. However, the antibiotics may hinder the diagnosis by masking the symptoms. A thorough history, including contact with any infected persons, exposure to pets or animals, history of travel, insect bites, unusual diet, may give clues to the origin of the fever.

NAET HELP

Emergency NAET on causative agent.

Collect a sample of child's saliva and treat with NAET; if the disease has already progressed, then treat a sample of urine, body secretion, sweat, blood, or stool. In the case of fever of unknown origin, please check every item the child is eating, drinking, inhaling and touching.

Treat for NAET group-A. Then treat by priority.

Collect a sample of daily food & drinks and treat using child-help protocol until the symptoms get better.

ACUHELP: Massage LI-11 for 1 minute counterclockwise as needed to reduce the fever.

Supplements

Calcium lactate 1 pill every two hours for five times during the day to reduce fever.

Agastache formula 1/2 gram twice a day.

Vitamin C, vitamin B, vitamin A, and trace minerals, after clearing the allergy.

Fresh ginger tea, one ounce twice daily after meals. This herb helps to balance the stomach, reduces the fever, stabilizes the whole energy of the body. A very useful herb used in a variety of conditions with good results.

Allergy to Rice

Six-year-old Cindy ran a continuous fever for three months. Her temperature remained between 102-103 degrees. She did not have any complaints of runny nose, sore throat, visible eruptions on the body. She appeared lethargic and listless. She was placed on antibiotics by her pediatrician for over a month without any reduction in her fever. Mother's sister, a herbalist gave her different herbs that also didn't work on her fever. Her WBC (white blood cell) was slightly raised on the blood test. She was diagnosed as having "fever of unknown origin." Finally her mother began giving her baby aspirin 1 every four hours and it kept the temperature down. She had to give the pill every 4 hours, otherwise her temperature reached the previous level. She was referred to us by one of the mothers of Cindy's classmate. We tested her by NTT and found that she was eating a special rice that was the cause of her fever. Her mother had bought a 50 lbs bag of rice and for the last three months she was fed on that rice everyday since the pudding made from rice, sugar and cinnamon was one of Cindy's favorite foods. She was treated for that particular rice using NAET. Her temperature dropped to normal after 24 hours from the initial treatment and maintained normal ever since.

Allergic Rhinitis

Seasonal or perennial sneezing, nasal congestion, runny nose, and often conjunctivitis characterize allergic rhinitis. Fifteen percent of the population, both adults and children, suffer from allergic rhinitis. It can be seasonal or perennial. Seasonal allergic rhinitis is usually caused by sensitivities to pollens from trees, grasses, weeds or airborne spores, which are present in the spring, summer and/or early fall. Year round symptoms, perennial allergic rhinitis is generally caused by sensitivity to house dust, dust mites, animal dander and mold spores. Food and chemical allergies (mainly sugars, minerals, banana, and detergent) can also cause perennial nasal symptoms. NAET treatments can give great relief in most cases.

NAET HELP

Emergency NAET on the causative agent if found.

Treat using child-help protocol for nasal discharge.

Then treat the NAET group-A, pollens, dust, and grass; then treat by priority for the rest of the classic NAET group.

Collect a sample of daily food and treat with NAET.

ACUHELP: Massage LI-4 1-3 minutes three times a day.

Supplements

Anise-seed-steam inhalations to reduce nasal congestion.

Allerplex one capsule, once or twice daily.

Parotid 1 pill twice a day.

Minor Blue Dragon formula 1/2 capsule twice daily.

Multivitamin 1 daily

My Son's Asthma

My four year old son was in one of his extreme asthmatic attacks, even using his facial muscles to breathe—this after just having spent two hours on a hospital inhaler. Dr. Devi had me listen to his distressed lungs through a stethoscope and it was frightening! A few moments after one NAET treatment for water chemicals we listened to his lungs again—and they were perfectly normal!

Vone Deporter
Woodland Hills, CA

Hay Fever

Hay fever is the acute form of allergic rhinitis. Wind-borne pollens generally induce it. The spring type is due to tree pollens (elm, oak, birch, and olive); the summer type due to grass pollens (Bermuda) and to weed pollens (Russian thistle); and the fall type due to weed pollens (ragweed). The nose, roof of the mouth, pharynx, and eyes begin to itch after the pollen season begins. Sneezing, frontal headaches and irritability may occur. Conjunctivitis, coughing and wheezing may develop as the season progresses. Sometimes foods and drinks also can give symptoms of hay-fever.

NAET HELP

Emergency NAET on the causative agent.

Treat the classic NAET group.

ACUHELP: Massage LI-4 for 1 minute three times daily.

Supplements

Allerplex one capsule, once or twice daily.

Antronex one tablet every two hours until the symptoms are diminished.

Minor blue dragon formula 1 capsule twice daily.

Vitamin C, Vitamin B, vitamin A, and Trace minerals.

The Greens moved to Southern California from Chicago in time for the new school year to begin. Everyone in the family was excited. The winters were long in Chicago and the children were looking forward to playing outside all year long. The family enjoyed going to the beaches, parks and mountains on the weekends. The boys joined soccer teams and spent as much time outside as possible. Their mother noticed that the two oldest boys would rub their eyes and complain that their eyes itched. They began breathing through their mouths more and more. The youngest boy's nasal passages were always blocked. By the end of the school year their symptoms had become chronic. Ron, the youngest boy developed a nasal twang to his voice. When they came to the clinic the two older boys had liquid in their ears and complained of earaches. Muscle testing indicated that they were allergic to pollens, trees, grasses, flowers and molds as well as many foods, including sugar, corn , wheat, and beans. After being treated for the basic ten food groups and environmental allergens their hay-fever and allergic rhinitis were completely eliminated. They are now back to enjoying the outdoors.

Bronchitis

This is an inflammation of the tracheobronchial tree, may be mild, can become serious, infectious or chronic. Airflow obstruction is a problem and pneumonia can develop. It often begins as an upper respiratory infection: slight fever, malaise, chills, back and muscle pain, and sore throat. The beginning of a distressing cough usually signals the start of bronchitis. Bed rest until the fever subsides is usually recommended along with plenty of fluids.

NAET HELP

Emergency NAET on the causative agent.

Cinnamon tea to reduce chest congestion.

Cumin tea 1 ounce twice a day to reduce cough.

Treat the child's saliva using child-help protocol at the first sign of the disease; if the disease has already progressed, then treat a sample of urine, body secretion, sputum, sweat, blood, and/ or stool.

Then treat the classic NAET groups.

In the case of a bronchitis, please check every item the child is eating, drinking, inhaling and touching for possible allergies, if found, treat with NAET for the item.

ACUHELP: Massage LI-11 and Lu-7 bilateral for 1-3 minutes each four times a day.

Supplements

Calcium lactate may be used one tablet every 2 hours for 5 times a day with water to reduce fever; reduce to one tablet twice daily after stabilizing the fever.

Vitamin C, Vitamin B, vitamin A, trace minerals, may be given.

Agastache formula one capsule once or twice a day.

Minor Bupluerum 1/2 Capsule twice daily for 2 weeks. Then evaluate the condition with your doctor.

Drenamin 1 pill three times a day.

Allergy to Shellfish

Sarah was six-years-old when her parents brought her to our clinic with the history of frequent bronchitis, walking pneumonia and asthma. She used an inhaler everyday and slept with three pillows and a humidifier every night to help her breathe. She couldn't participate in any physical activities in school. Her parents had taken her to their family doctor, a pediatrician, a conventional allergist to give her some relief. They eliminated all the indoor plants, carpeting and stuffed animals from her room, but her throat would still close up and she would break out in hives periodically. Several times she had to be hospitalized. She was missing so much school that the teacher told her parents she might have to repeat the first grade. Her mother brought her to our clinic after talking to one of our patient's mothers whose son was Sarah's classmate. Sarah was allergic to all the basic 15 food groups as well as environmental and chemical allergens; however, after she was treated for fish and shellfish she no longer had difficulty breathing and the hives on her body disappeared. Her mother had been trying to eat less meat to lower her cholesterol and served fish two to three times a week. She was giving Sarah tuna fish for lunch on a regular basis. She no longer needs an inhaler, humidifier or three pillows at night to sleep with. The best news of all is that she was promoted to second grade and is running and jumping happily in the playground.

Common Cold

Common cold may be caused by any substance: foods, drinks, household dust, cosmetics, household pets, animal dander, chalk, newspaper ink, paint, plastics, chemical sprays, molds, soaps, perfumes and other chemical agents.

Rami, was three-years-old when he started getting colds. His nose was always running and his eyes were watery. His mother had enrolled him in pre-school and thought he must be catching colds from the other children. Rami never wanted to stay home from preschool. He loved to finger paint and write on the chalkboard. He would bring home his artwork and his mother would hang it proudly on the refrigerator. His nasal passages and ears were becoming so congested that the doctor thought it would be best to insert tubes in his ears. He would wake up crying at night from the pain in his ears. After examining him, I found him to be allergic to the finger paint, and newsprint and chalk he was using everyday in school. After clearing for these items his nasal passages and earaches cleared. He was lucky he didn't need to have tubes inserted in his ears.

NAET HELP

Emergency NAET on the causative agent.
Anise seed tea 1 ounce twice a day for congestion.

Fresh ginger tea 1 ounce after meals for digestion.
Child-help NAEt on nasal discharge at the first sign of the disease.
Then treat for NAET group-A
Collect a sample of daily foods and drinks and do child-help NAET daily.
ACUHELP: Massage LI-4 1-3 minutes three times a day.

Supplements

Calcium lactate may be given one tablet every two hours for 5 times a day to reduce fever; reduce to one tablet twice daily after stabilizing the fever.
Vitamin C, Vitamin B, vitamin A, trace minerals, may be given.
Agastache formula one capsule with water twice daily.
Drenamin 1 pill three times a day.

Can Vitamin C Cause or Cure a Cold?

I was giving chewable vitamin C 500 milligrams daily to my 7 year old son to prevent him from getting colds. It seemed that he would get a cold once or twice a week and was still taking 500 units of vitamin C tablets a day. She found out that my son was allergic to vitamin C, he got treated and now he hasn't had a cold for more than a year. I continue to give him vitamin C. Now he can absorb it.

Maria M. , Buena Park, CA

Asthma

Asthma is a chronic inflammatory disorder of the lungs characterized by episodic and reversible symptoms of airflow obstruction and increased airway responsiveness to a variety of stimuli. According to one of the surveys released by CDC (Center for Disease Control), in 1998, nearly 17 million Americans had asthma and the prevalence rate has increased by 75 percent between 1980 and 1994. In addition, the survey also found that nearly four out of five Americans (77 percent) are directly affected by asthma. In 1998, asthma affected an estimated 17,299,000 persons in the United States. The state with the largest estimated number of persons with asthma was California (2,268,300), followed by New York (1,236,200).

Asthma is the ninth leading cause of hospitalization nationally. In 1998, an estimated six million Americans were hospitalized, treated in emergency rooms or required urgent care for asthma. The finding is one of several that suggest that nation is falling far short of new government guidelines for asthma care, and that for many people, a generally controllable disease may be out of control. The death rate from asthma increased by 40% in 1998 from the previous survey of 1994; it was five times higher for blacks than whites.

Asthma is the leading cause of hospitalization for children and the number one chronic condition causing school absenteeism. In 1998, 49 percent of children with asthma missed school due to asthma. Another survey estimated that over 2 billion dollars were spent in hospital care and the total cost of asthma care was over six billion dollars. The frequency and severity of the symptoms vary greatly from person to person.

What are the common triggers of asthma?

Allergy to Food, drinks, vitamins, food additives, and drugs. Environmental allergens: house dust, dust mites, industrial dust, mold, pollen, grass, weeds, animal dander, and animal epithelial.

- Air pollutants: cigarette smoke, auto exhaust, smog, chemicals, infections in the respiratory tract.

- Weather changes: cold, heat, humidity, fog, dampness, damp heat and damp cold.

- Exercise.

- Emotional factors.

Sulfites are widely publicized substances that have been added as a preservative to salads and potatoes in restaurant salad bars and in the fast food industry. The intention was to maintain freshness (or at least the appearance of freshness and flavor) as these vegetables sit out in display cases for long periods of time. Unfortunately, sulfites are salt derivatives of sulfuric acid, which many asthma sufferers are highly allergic to.

NAET HELP

Treat for the causative agent.

Treat NAET group-A first. Then treat using priority if the asthma is still not gone by then. In most cases, within 13 treatments, remarkable changes will be noticed in their frequency, and intensity. A few children may continue to get asthma with the contacts with environmental substances like chemicals, plastics, latex, automobile fumes, fabrics, school work materials, coloring agents, pens, marker inks, colored books, etc.

ACUHELP: Massage Lung-7 as needed.

Supplements

Agastache formula one capsule twice daily.

Minor blue dragon formula 1/2 capsule twice daily

Hoelen and schizandra 1 capsule twice daily for 1 year

Betaine HCL 1 with each meal

Vitamin C, Vitamin B, vitamin A, and trace minerals

Fresh ginger tea 1 ounce twice a day after meals

After NAET group A, collect a small portion of each meal in a test tube and self treat every night. (Instruction for self-treatment is given in Chapter 9).

Bronchial Asthma & Body ache

For approximately 15 years ever since I was a child I have suffered with frequent colds which turn into extended bouts with bronchial asthma and extreme weakness and fatigue. The doctors treated me with extensive doses of antibiotics, steroids, antihistamines, and cough medicine. I was usually depressed and so weak I could hardly move out of bed and I had to get shots every day for weeks. Along with it my stomach would gurgle and hurt for the duration of the medication. The doctors thought the stomach problems were due to steroids.

One night I had the flu and started wheezing, so I took some of the cough medicine I used to take. I had not had a cold since I moved out of Louisiana's humid climate, but I still had some of my old cough medicine. One hour later, I awoke aching all over, with my stomach hurting and gurgling. I called Dr. Devi and she told me to bring the cough medicine. As soon as she treated me for it I got my strength back, was no longer depressed and my stomach felt normal.

For years, I had severe body pain, and headaches. My pains left for good when I completed treatments for classic NAET groups.

Carole W., Irvine, CA

An Allergy to City Water

A four-year-old boy had been suffering from severe asthmatic attacks since he was an infant. His mother had tried everything from herbal remedies to conventional allergy treatments. He was given inhalers, steroids, special bedding, air purifiers, and injections to desensitize him to molds, pollens, dust mites, etc., but he ended up in the emergency room at least once a month. He would spend 2-3 hours on an inhaler before his lungs were clear enough for him to breathe by himself. His parents were constantly monitoring him, never wanting to leave him alone. They limited his play time and kept him on a restricted diet. By the time he was brought to the clinic, Doug was pale, weak and had so much difficulty breathing that he was using his facial muscles to help him breathe. I listened to his lungs through a stethoscope and they were totally filled with liquid. When I let his mother listen she grew pale. After muscle testing, he was found to be allergic to the chemicals in the water he was drinking daily. After treating him for the chemicals in drinking water I let his mother listen to his chest again. His lungs were perfectly clear! He hasn't had any difficulty breathing since. He plays, eats, drinks and looks as healthy as all his friends at his preschool now. City water has been found to be a culprit in a number of childhhood asthmatic cases in my office. City water should not be used for drinking without boiling, filtering or purification, especially in Southern California.

Asthma and Sinusitis

I came to Dr. Devi through a friend in 1985. I suffered from asthma since childhood. During the last 7 years I developed severe sinusitis. I was on antibiotics at least 20 days of a month. My symptoms were sinus headaches, shortness of breath, coughing and wheezing. Within the first two months, my sinus headaches were reduced by 90 percent. By then the coughing and wheezing were virtually gone. I was treated by NAET for 8 months and I was completely free of symptoms. Previously I tested positive for grasses, pollens and trees. As per her advice I waited for 10 months more after completion of NAET to do a traditional allergy testing (RAST). I tested negative for grasses, pollens and trees this time. I am free of asthma and sinusitis for the past 14 years! Thanks to Dr. Devi and NAET.

Greg A., Anaheim, CA

Cough

What are the common triggers of cough?

• Allergy to Food, drinks, vitamins, food additives, drugs and environmental agents like pesticides, detergents, dust, animal dander, etc.

• Air pollutants: cigarette smoke, auto exhaust, smog, chemicals, infections in the respiratory tract.

• Weather changes: cold, heat, humidity, fog, dampness, damp heat and damp cold.

• Emotional factors.

NAET HELP

Emergency NAET on the causative agent.

Anise seed tea 1 ounce three times a day.

Treat for the causative agent for an acute attack. If it is not an acute attack, you should follow the normal NAET protocol--that is to treat NAET group-A first. After treating with NAET group-A, you can prioritize the treatments if the cough is still not gone by then. In most cases, within 13 treatments, remarkable changes will be noticed in their frequency, and intensity.

After treating for group-A, collect a small portion of each meal in a test tube and self treat every night.

ACUHELP: Massage Lung-7 as needed.

Supplements

Hoelen and schizandra (from lotus herbs) 1 capsule twice daily for 1 year.

Betaine HCL 1 with each meal.

Vitamin C, Vitamin B, vitamin A, and trace minerals.

Drenamin 1 pill three times a day.

Allergy to Cough Medicine

7-year-old Justin seemed to be sick with colds, cough and sinusitis all the time for a year now. He suffered from constant sinus congestion. His sinus congestion would turn into long spells of coughs in bed with excessive mucous production. The pediatrician recommended a special cough medicine. Soon after taking the medication, some nights he would start to wheeze and he would cry saying that his stomach hurts. The doctor changed the medication, but nothing helped. His mother kept him home from preschool isolating him from children of his age in an attempt to keep him from getting sick. His constant cough and flu-like symptoms continued. He was beginning to have asthma on and off through the day by the time his mother found out about NAET from one of her church members.

We tested him on our special computer for his allergies. He had moderate allergies to most foods and drinks. He was moderately allergic to the NAET group-A, but not high enough to produce the problem he was suffering. We tested him through NTT and found he was allergic to the mattress where he slept every night. We asked the parents to bring a piece of his mattress. He was very allergic to the mattress. That was the culprit in his case to cause sinus congestion, cough and finally asthma. He was also allergic to the cough medicine. Because of his allergy to the medicine he did not get any relief by taking it; in fact his symptoms got worse. If the pediatrician was aware of NAET testing procedures, he would have prescribed a nonallergic medicine to him and it should have helped to control his symptoms. After passing the treatment for mattress (which had to be treated three times) and cough medicine (which had to be treated two times) his constant colds and flu-like symptoms disappeared along with his stomach ache.

Insomnia

Many children suffer from insomnia and night-crying. They may be suffering from simple allergies to the foods, clothes, blankets or crib toys. Another reason they would have problem is due to underfeeding. They may be just hungry or thirsty. They may be growing fast and the quantity of the food may not be sufficient.

NAET HELP

Emergency NAET on the causative agent.

Check all the recent foods and drinks. Check for all new clothes and chemicals used earlier in the day.

Try to treat for NAET group-A.

Treat iron mix, spleen, and combinations.

Puree one or two dates and feed the child daily.

ACUHELP: Massage HT-7 and GV-20 for a minute, two-three times a day.

Allergy to Woolen Blanket

Rachel, a new patient at our clinic, brought her 5-month-old son in for me to see. She was very distraught because for months (a week or so after she brought him from the hospital) she wasn't able to keep her son from crying all night long. He would only fall asleep if she held him in her arms. Her husband said she was spoiling him and should just let him cry, but the baby was having difficulty breathing. She could hear him wheezing and his lungs were congested. His pediatrician couldn't find anything wrong with the infant. The weather was cold all along and he was given a beautiful woolen blanket as gift that she put on the baby to keep him warm at night. She only used it when the baby was in his crib. After testing the baby through his mother (as a surrogate) we discovered that he was allergic to the woolen blanket. After he was treated for the blanket (through his mother), both the mother and baby began sleeping peacefully through the night.

Allergy to Fireplace Smoke

Deena, 8 years old, developed sinusitis and asthma every fall and winter. Her doctors prescribed antibiotics and inhalers for her. Her symptoms would last until the weather turned warm. She was constantly wheezing and coughing. Her sinus headaches made it difficult for her to complete her homework or study and she began getting poor grades in school. Through muscle testing we found that it was something she was breathing in her house that was giving her respiratory problems. Her mother thought of all the things she was using in the house, but everything tested fine. Then she said that when the weather gets cool she loves to put the fire on at the fireplace in the family room/kitchen area where the family spends most of its time. Deena tested highly allergic to fireplace smoke. She spent most of the time sitting by the fireplace in the fall and winter doing her homework, watching TV, and eating dinner. The fireplace smoke was causing her asthma and sinusitis. Now that she has passed her treatment for fireplace smoke, not only is her asthma and sinusitis gone, but she also is a straight A student!

Allergy to Damp Air

Jason and his family loved sailing and lived near the ocean. His older brother would get up early in the morning to surf before he went to school. His father would take the family to Catalina for the weekends. Everyone looked forward to going on the sailboat. Jason would usually return from his sailboat trips with a cough and/or an asthma. Many times his inhaler wasn't enough and he would need steroids to clear his lungs. We tested him and found he was highly allergic to the damp air, mold, salt and wind. After being treated for these items and their combinations he enjoys his sails without cough or asthma.

Fear Triggered His Asthma

Every Saturday my seven year old son suffered from asthma. Medication or sprays did not help him at all. I had to take him to the emergency room. Just by sitting in the emergency room waiting area, his asthma would go away. Saturday was his father's turn to take him for the weekend. Since he did not feel well on Saturday evenings, he could not go with him. When I brought him to Dr. Devi, she found out that the cause of his asthma was an emotional issue. He was afraid to go with his father because he would have to spend the night in his room with his gay roommate; so he began having asthmatic episodes, spending Saturday evening in the emergency room. Then Sunday, his father would take him out for a couple of hours.

*After he was treated for his allergy and fear of his father's room-
mate, he stopped having Saturday night asthma.*
   Belle Cole, Fullerton, CA

Allergy to Perfume

Angela, a patient of ours, would leave her 6-month-old baby
at her mother's once a week when she came for a treatment. Whenever she picked the baby up from her mother's house, the little
girl would be wheezing and having difficulty breathing. Her mother
would tell her that whenever she tried to comfort the baby and
held her in her arms she cried and cried. Through muscle testing I
traced the problem to something the grandmother was wearing.
Angela brought her daughter and mother with her on her next
visit to the clinic. The grandmother was asked to wear everything
she wore the last time she was with the baby. We tested the baby
through her mother. There was no reaction to any of the
grandmother's clothing or jewelry. We put the baby in the
grandmother's arms and the baby immediately started to wheeze.
The grandmother's perfume was causing the asthmatic symptoms.
We quickly treated the infant (through the mother) for that particular perfume and baby and grandmother enjoy each other's company now without any negative reactions.

Sinus Headaches and Allergic Rhinitis
*I came to Doctor Devi a year ago with sinus headaches,
shortness of breath, coughing, runny nose and wheezing. Within
the first two months, my sinus headaches were reduced almost
by 90 percent. The coughing and wheezing are virtually all gone.
Now, we are working on eliminating allergy symptoms. I have
been very pleased with her treatment and I have recommended
her to many others.*
   Jim Ashley, Anaheim

Allergens like pollens, flowers, molds and dusts most often cause asthma in asthma sufferers. In addition, asthma can be caused by allergies to almost any: food, clothing, chemicals, perfumes, synthetic substances and natural substances. Cold, heat, dampness and moisture can cause an asthmatic reaction as well as an allergy to one's spouse, children or another human associate or even a pet.

Allergy to Grasses and Pollens

Matt was a husky 9-year-old, who loved sports. His parents signed him up for Little League baseball. He was always the first boy on the field ready to play. But baseball season always found him with coughs, sinus problems, and recently his asthmatic symptoms were getting more severe. His family doctor told him that he shouldn't be playing baseball regularly. Matt became depressed and wouldn't leave his room when his parents agreed with the doctor to take him off the team. Another Little League parent, whose child was a patient of ours, referred them to us. We tested him and found he was allergic to pollens, grasses, trees, molds and fungus. He began regular visits and after 20 treatments his cough, sinus and asthma difficulties have been completely eliminated. Matt received a trophy this season for being the best pitcher on his team.

Allergy to Socks and Shoes

9 year old David, could not play his little league game without falling on the grass at least three or four times a day. He was falling frequently in the school for no reason. Finally he was excluded from the game. He was very sad. His mother brought him to the office to check his back after one of those falls in the school. After checking him, listening his story I tested him for his socks and shoes. He tested highly allergic to them. Immediately he was treated for his socks and shoes and sent home with slippers. Next day he was tested and he passed the treatments for the socks and shoes. Two weeks later, he returned to the office to report that he was back in the little league and hasn't fallen down ever since the treatment for the socks and shoes.

Peanut Allergy

My eight year old son had severe peanut allergy ever since he was a baby. When he was three years old he had to be taken to the emergency room after he ate a touch of peanut butter. He would get asthma, break out in huge hives and his throat would swell if he smelled peanut oil or roasted peanuts. So we never used peanuts or peanut oil in the house. It was a nightmare for me to read all the labels before I buy food products or send him to school where children eat peanuts and candies and most of them included peanuts. Then I heard about NAET. Sam was treated by NAET for peanuts. After he was treated he accidently ate a cookie with peanut. He did not have a reaction. I am not planning to feed him peanuts for meals. But I am more at ease now knowing that he will not have a life-threatening reaction if he ate peanuts accidently somewhere.

Thank you Dr Devi, for your miraculous contribution to the world!

Sharon M., LongBeach, CA

Food colorings cause a lot of problems including respiratory problems, skin disorders, hyperactivity, autism, learning disability and neurological disorders among young ones.

Allergy to Food Coloring

Four-year-old Kate loved to help her mother in the kitchen. She especially likes to make cookies and Jell-O. Her mother delighted in seeing Kate decorate the cookies with colored sprinkles and icing. They would shape the Jell-O with cookie cutters into animal shapes and create stories about them. It was their special time together. But for the last few months Kate had been getting colds and the medication the doctor prescribed for her congestion and difficult breathing wasn't helping. She began staying in bed later and later each morning. She would cough through the night. She was too sick to play with her friends. When she was brought to our clinic she was very pale with dark circles under her eyes, wheezing and coughing every time she tried to talk. After being treated for the NAET group-A, her cough subsided and she was much more energetic. It wasn't until she was treated for food colorings that her symptoms subsided completely. The red, green, and blue food colorings used in the icing to decorate the cookies and the cherry Jell-O she loved to eat were the causes of her asthmatic symptoms. After passing her treatment for food coloring she ran into my office the following week with a big smile on her face and handed me the cookies she decorated.

Tomato Induced Asthma!

I used to get a severe asthma and sinusitis whenever I ate tomatoes or anything made with tomatoes. Spaghetti with basil and garlic sauce was my favorite. Every time I ate that I used to get my throat tight, and in another few minutes, I would begin to get asthma. After I was treated for tomatoes by Dr. Devi, I no longer get any reactions after I eat tomatoes.

Jean Trott, Anaheim

Allergy to milk products

Seema was an active fifth grader, always running, biking or playing tennis and taking ballet lessons. Her mother was constantly driving her from one activity to the next. She could barely keep up with her daughter's schedule. She was worried about her daughter getting enough nutritious food on such a hectic schedule. So she made sure Seema would get enough calcium by bringing along a snack after school: milk with cheese and fruit, yogurt and granola, vanilla or chocolate pudding, and sometimes a treat of ice cream or frozen yogurt. After ballet lessons she noticed that her daughter was having difficulty breathing. Seema complained that her throat hurt. Her mother kept Seema home from school and curtailed all her activities for a week. Her symptoms cleared, so she resumed her normal schedule again. After tennis Seema began coughing and coughed through the night. The next day she was so congested her mother took her to the doctor. After examining Seema he told her mother that she had exercise-induced asthma. He recommended that Seema stop all physical activities and prescribed an inhaler for her and a steroid medication. Seema became very depressed sitting at home after school so her mother would always have a special treat for a snack for her. By late afternoon each day Seema would begin to cough and become very tired, her mother became very concerned. Her neighbor was one of our patients and suggested that she make an appointment to see us. After testing Seema we found that she was highly allergic to milk, milk products, cheese and yogurt - all the food items her mother thought would be the healthiest for her to eat. After Seema cleared for the milk products, cheese and yogurt, her symptoms subsided and she returned to all her after- school activities. She no longer needs an inhaler or any medications.

Pneumonia

In the USA, about 2 million people develop pneumonia each year and 40,000 to 70,000 people die; it ranks sixth among all the diseases as a cause of death and is the most common lethal infection. Typical symptoms include cough, fever, and sputum production. Neonatal pneumonia occurs many times after complications occur during pregnancy (premature labor or a difficult forceps delivery). Antibiotics should be used judiciously because they may be harmful to the infant's flora. Signs and symptoms of pneumonia include: cough and fever, chest pain, headache, chills, rapid heart rate, rapid breathing, shortness of breath, dark or bloody sputum, bluish discoloration around the eyes, lips, and nail beds.

NAET HELP

Treat for the causative agent if found.

Collect a sample of child's saliva at the first sign of the disease and treat with NAET.

If the disease has already progressed, then treat a sample of urine, sputum, body secretion, sweat, blood, or stool.

Treat with NAET group-A, then treat by priority.

ACUHELP: Massage Lung-1, Lung-7 bilaterally three times a day.

Supplements

Allerplex 1 twice daily as needed to reduce the allergic symptoms.

Agastache formula one capsule once or twice daily for children between 2-10 years of age.

Minor blue dragon formula 1-2 twice daily for minor asthma.

Minor Bupluerum formula 1 capsule twice daily.

Vitamin C, vitamin B, vitamin A, and trace minerals.

Viral Meningitis

Headache, pain, stiffness in the neck and back, and muscular aches with fever, malaise, anorexia, and vomiting are symptoms of meningitis. Meningitis is an inflammation of the membranes of the brain or spinal cord usually caused by bacteria, viruses, fungi, and rarely parasites. It can result in death, seizures, deafness, and other serious neurological consequences. Contacting viral meningitis during the first four weeks of life can be fatal. 85% of viral meningitis cases occur in outbreaks in the summer and early fall. 80% of most bacterial meningitis occur in patients less than 2 years old. Meningitis caused by candida (fungus) occurs in premature infants and others with impaired immune systems. Lasting effects of the infection may occur in up to 25% of children who contact the illness.

NAET HELP

Treat for the causative agent if found.

Collect a sample of child's saliva at the first sign of the disease and treat with NAET.

If the disease has already progressed, then treat a sample of urine, body secretion, sweat, blood, or stool.

Treat city water, drinking water, milk, any prepackaged food you bought at the store, and any unusual food your child ate lately. Check your drinking water source and city water supply if you have an epidemic of viral infection in your area. Boil the water in an open container for 20 minutes and cool it before you use for drinking purposes during an epidemic.

Treat NAET group-A.

Cumin tea 1 ounce twice a day.

ACUHELP: LI-4 and Lung-1 bilaterally for 1-3 minutes three times a day.

Supplements

Allerplex 1 twice daily.

Calcium lactate 1 every six hours.

Vitamin C, Vitamin B, vitamin A, Trace minerals, antioxidants may be given.

Agastache formula one capsule once or twice daily for children between 2-10 years of age.

Parotid 1 pill three times a day.

Drenamin 1 pill three times a day.

Apple cider vinegar 1 drops in 1 ounce of boiled cooled water, with sugar or honey to taste, one ounce every two hours.

Gastrointestinal Problems

This group of problems are the ones you encounter most frequently among little children. There are three major functions predominating all other functions in the body: Digestion, assimilation and elimination. Children rarely get sick if these three functions run smoothly. The problems begin if any disturbance happens to these functions.

Although all types of gastro intestinal (GI) tract allergies are usually caused by food, some other substances: inhalants, fabrics like nylons, flannels, wool, rubber, latex products, plastics, formaldehyde, etc., may also be responsible for this condition. Usually milk is the greatest offender, and most of these children are sensitive to milk products. Other foods include peanuts and shellfish.

Allergens can cause indigestion, vomiting, abdominal pains, flatulence, celiac sprue, leaky gut syndrome, Crohn's disease, and ulcerative colitis, etc. In ulcerative colitis, probably a sore-like canker occurs at the site of a small lesion in the intestines and then becomes infected. When this occurs, a very large and excruciatingly painful ulcer develops.

Nausea

Any allergen can cause nausea. Lack of digestive enzymes, stomach acids, allergy to the digestive juices causing poor digestion, overeating, viral or bacterial infections, parasites, growths or tumors, lack of nutrients, are some of the causes of nausea. Lack of hydrochloric acid production or production of abnormal hydrochloric acids in the stomach can cause nausea. Emotional upsets produce nausea in many children.

NAET HELP
Treat for the causative agent if found.
Treat for NAET group-A. Then treat by priority.
Fresh ginger slices, ginger preserve, or ginger candy to chew.
Cold fresh ginger tea a few sips at a time might help.
ACUHELP: Massage PC-6 for 1-3 minutes as needed.

Supplements
Agastache formula one capsule once or twice daily for children between 2-10 years of age.
Betaine HCL 1 pill, twice daily.
Multizyme 1/2 twice a day with meals.
Apple cider vinegar 1 drop in an ounce of water with sugar or honey to taste, give one ounce every two hours until the nausea subsides.
Ginger Ale one ounce every two hours

Peanut Anaphylaxis

Our daughter Haarnoor and son Nausher had an allergy to peanut butter and had been to the emergency room several times. Just from the smell of it they had been in the hospital. We are not only thankful to Dr. Nambudripad but indebted to her. Today both our daughter and son had peanuts and had no allergic reaction. If there is any way we can be of any help or if anyone wants to call us, we will be more than happy to support and sign documents to prove it.

Sincerely,

Jumesh and Geetika Walia, Studio City, CA

jumeshwalia@hotmail.com

No more Allergies to Milk or Milk Products!

As a small child, our son Andrew was sickly. He had tubes surgically inserted in his ears at age 4. Soon afterward he developed problems when he ate foods containing milk or chocolate. Andrew threw up his food, then was ravenously hungry afterward. Sometimes Andrew would suffer excruciating headaches as well.

After many NAET treatments, Andrew began to improve. He was treated for the NAET group-A, chocolate, Caffeine, milk, cheese, meat mix, heat, amino acids, leather and with many combinations.

Now Andrew is a healthy thirteen-year-old teenager, suffering an occasional headache instead of several headaches per week. I am cooking with regular milk now instead of rice milk and Andrew seems to tolerate it well.

Thank you, Dr. Devi, for your unfailing enthusiasm, which is apparent in your book, Say Good-bye to Illness. I know many families such as ours will be able to eat and function normally.

Karen Hyatt
Monroe, North Carolina

Milk Allergy

If your child is allergic to milk and milk products, it is very frustrating news. Milk is the easiest food you can provide your child. Almost every regular prepackaged food product in the market contains milk. NAET has been a blessing for milk allergy sufferers.

Homogenized milk also causes concern for many patients in the United States. Even after they are clear for the milk allergy, milk drinkers face an allergic reaction once in a while depending mainly on what the cattle are fed. Dairies have no control over what the cows are fed every day. Most nut-oil companies, after extracting the oils, dry the leftovers into compact cakes and sell them to the dairies, where they are randomly fed to the cows. When the cows secrete milk, some of the substances from the nuts are also secreted through the milk. Sometimes, if the cows are fed with hay and grasses that have been sprayed with pesticides, these substances will also be excreted in the milk.

If you have allergic tendencies, you can react at anytime when you drink milk. The particular reaction is not due to an allergy to milk, but to the pesticides or other ingredients in the milk sample. This should be kept in mind when treating for milk allergy.

I am Not Allergic to Milk Any More!

Hello Mala & Mohan,

How are you? I feel great, thanks to you. Yesterday, Friday, 8/25/00 like a little kid with a new toy, I had to try out any food containing lactose to test myself. I had my opportunity at the San Diego Zoo — I had a small portion of ice cream. Then the countdown began, from 20 minutes. Then 19, 18, 17, 16, and so on. Zero - nothing. I had no reaction!! I waited another 20 minutes. Still, no reaction. So I had a little more ice cream. One hour, two hours, three hours later, still no reaction. Amazing!! Later on for dinner I had some milk chocolate. Still no reaction! NAET is the best thing that's happened to me. I feel like I have a renewed Life!

With much appreciation,
Tom Moy

Allergy occurs with considerable frequency in the intestines, usually causing symptoms of colic, cramping, constipation, diarrhea, soreness, and bleeding of the intestinal walls (as in irritable bowel syndrome, celiac sprue, Crohn's disease, etc.). Severe pain may result from allergies to various every-day food products such as wheat, grains, milk, corn, spices, fats, beans, proteins, meat, parasites, etc. or it could be from an obstruction in the intestines by edema (swelling) of these organs. Intestinal allergy patients frequently have a tendency to bleed in various parts of the body as in the case of a girl who had nosebleeds, bleeding from the rectum, or hemorrhaging of the conjunctiva (bloodshot eyes) whenever she drank milk.

When your milk allergy produces constipation, it may cause the intestines to retain the fecal matter (unabsorbed residues of intestinal excretions) until it is putrefied, causing intermittent attacks of constipation, flatulence and diarrhea. In some cases, milk causes such severe diarrhea that even a few drops are sufficient to bring on an attack.

Thrush / Candida

Thrush is a candida infection inside the mouth. The creamy white patches cling to the tongue and sometimes on the sides of the mouth. This can be painful too. The patches can be scraped off easily with a finger or a spoon. The use of antibiotics can cause thrush in some children. Antibiotics kill off the friendly bacteria from the intestines and this could increase the chance of getting Thrush (also called, candidiasis, moniliasis).

Allergy to yeast producing food products can encourage yeast and candida growth in the system. Lack of hydrochloric acid in the system also can cause overgrowth of candida or thrush.

NAET HELP

Treat for the causative agent. Treat a sample of child's saliva at the first sign of the disease.

If the disease has already progressed, then treat a sample of urine, body secretion, sweat, blood, or stool.

Then NAET group-A. Then treat by priority.

Clean the tongue and mouth with diluted apple cider vinegar, lemon juice, or nutmeg tea.

Take extra care in cleaning the feeding bottles, nipples, pacifiers, etc.

Commonly seen allergens: Cow's milk, goat milk, mother's milk, soy milk, sugar products, milk products, yeast products, feeding bottles, rubber nipples, pacifiers, tethers, baby wipes, soap, detergent, plastic or rubber toys.

NAET treatments on yeast producing foods and chemicals have successfully eliminated thrush and systemic yeast/candida growth in many people. Check with your NAET practitioner for more detail.

ACUHELP: Massage St-36 for 1-3 minutes twice a day.

Supplements

Apple cider vinegar 1 drop to 1 ounce of water, and give an ounce every hour to improve the acidity in the stomach.

Allerplex 1/2 twice daily as needed to reduce the allergic symptoms.

Agastache formula 1/2 capsule once or twice daily to improve digestive functions.

Fibromyalgia

Fibromyalgia in young children is unheard of in the past. Everyone assumes young children have better immune systems. They run around so much they burn up the toxins produced by the allergens as they produce. But now-a-days, many young children complain of general body ache, chronic fatigue, and fibromyalgia. It must be due to the affect of the chemicals explosion we are facing lately.

Commonly seen symptoms: general body ache, pain in special parts of the body, groin pain, pain in the head, complaining of pain when pulling or moving the hair, small joint pain, burning pain in any area of the body, sensitivity of skin, unable to wear tight or rough clothes, pain on movements, pain in the morning to get up from the bed, able to snap or crack the joints easily and repeatedly, insomnia, fatigue, headaches, restless leg syndrome, bruising easily, irregular appetite (extreme hunger or poor appetite), crying spells, depression, anger, procrastination, hallucination seeing things, or feeling things on the body; some children would say that "something rubbed against me," "I felt something touched me,"etc. This may be due to the severity of their allergies resulting; in nerve endings becoming over sensitive even to a gush of air and they may feel as if someone touched them; unable to complete homework successfully, etc.

NAET HELP

Treat for the causative agent if found, may be apples, spices, salt, phosphorus, dried beans, sugar, chocolate, etc.

Treat the saliva, blood, urine, etc.

NAET basic group-A, malic acid, oxalic acid vitamin C groups, bioflavonoid, then by priority.

ACUHELP: Massage PC-6 for 30 seconds to a minute twice daily to reduce pain.

Supplements

Hibiscus tea 1 ounce twice a day.

Allerplex 1/2 twice daily as needed to reduce the allergic symptoms.

Agastache formula 1/2 capsule once or twice daily to improve digestive functions.

Siler and Platycodon formula 1 twice a day.

Persica and Rhubarb formula 1 twice a day.

Drenamin 1 pill three time a day.

Fibromyalgia

I suffered fibromyalgia for 7 years. I tried all the medicines known to man to get my severe pain under control. All the expensive pain medications and antiinflammatory medicines didn't help me. My parents took me to church every week. I couldn't go to church because the incense made me sick and often made ne faint. Also I felt severe pains when I was on my knees to pray. Then I found NAET. I was skeptic in the beginning. But NAET treatments began working on me. The biggest leap towards wellness started after I treated for dried bean mix, oxalic acid, and coffee. Now I am free of my fibromyalgia. Thank you Dr. Devi, I don't have enough words thank you for discovering NAET.

Ileen Thomas, Orange, CA.

Gastritis

An inflammation of the lining of the stomach, gastritis is the most common cause of bleeding in the upper gastrointestinal tract in children. Any part of the gastrointestinal tract exposed to acid-peptic juice can interact abnormally leading to irritation of the affected tissue. In the normal stomach of an adult, the concentration of hydrogen ions at maximal secretion is 3 million times greater than that of blood and tissues. The normal defense mechanism of the gastrointestinal tract has various ways to protect the lining of the stomach and intestine. Some of the natural protective mechanisms are: the mucosal barrier that protects the gastric mucosa from "autodigestion" by secreting a protective mucous barrier; and secretion of bicarbonate by the surface epithelial cells neutralizing the excess production of acid as and when needed to maintain a homeostatic environment. These defense mechanisms are provided in children too. The normal defense, repair and healing mechanisms of the mucosa can fail when disrupted by exogenous factors like infections, drugs, etc. When the defense does not work properly various digestive disorders can develop as in gastritis, regurgitation, projectile vomiting, hyperacidity, heartburn, ulcer, giving rise to symptoms including upper abdominal pain and tenderness (usually after meals), loss of appetite, vomiting, irritability, and weight loss. An infection (tuberculosis, Heliobactor pylori, parasites), stress, drugs (anti-inflammatory drugs, steroids), alcohol, smoke, food allergy/sensitivity and genetic factors can also cause the disruption of the defense mechanisms. According to researchers, first degree relative of stomach disorder (example: gastric ulcer) patients are three times as likely to develop ulcers as the general population, and a monozygotic twin has a 50% chance of developing ulcers or such disorders if the other twin is affected.

NAET treatment is very effective in treating allergy-related gastritis and other gastric disorders.

NAET HELP
NAET on the causative agent if found.
Collect a sample of child's saliva at the first sign of the disease and treat with NAET.
Treat a sample of vomit or spit from the child each time the child vomits or spits.
Collect a sample of daily food and treat at bed-time.
Treat with NAET group-A
Then treat for stomach acid, sodium bicarbonate, gastric mucosa, collagen, epithelial cells, steroids, alcohol, tobacco smoke, parts of GI tract, DNA/RNA, bacteria, heliobactor pylori, blood, immunization drugs, any other drugs taken by the child or the

mother during the period of breast feeding or any combinations of the above.

ACUHELP: Massage St-36 for 1-3 minutes twice daily.

Supplements

Agastache formula one capsule once or twice daily to improve digestive functions.

Cardamom and fennel formula 1 cap. twice daily.

Multizyme1/2 capsule with each meal.

Anaphylaxis due to Shellfish

I reacted severely to fish or fish products since childhood. Whenever I ate a minute portion of fish or shellfish, my throat closed up, I couldn't breathe, I could break out with huge hives all over my body and I ended up in the emergency room for hours with cortisone and other emergency drugs. On a few occasions, I had to be hospitalized for a few days. One of my friends, who was treated by Dr. Devi for his peanut allergy, suggested that I see her for my life-threatening fish allergy. I was curious about NAET. She treated me for all the basics before she treated me for fish groups. I had a severe reaction during the first treatment for fish. As soon as she placed the clear glass vial with the energy of fish in my hand, my hand swelled up and I broke out in red hives all over the body. I got up from the treatment table to reach for my adrenaline shot which I carried all the time with me. But she stopped me. She commanded me to turn over. She looked very confident. I obeyed her and she applied firm pressure on my back, up and down along the spine for a few times. When she finished applying the acupressure along my spine, she asked me to turn on my back. She tested my arm.

I was strong. She asked me how I was doing. I was breathing better than ever and my throat did not feel restricted anymore. I looked at my bare arms. Red rashes began fading away. This is magic, I thought. She was standing in front of me with that smile of confidence waiting for my answer. "Better," I said with a sigh of relief.

I had to have three combination treatments for fish (fish group, with lungs, colon, spleen and liver, fish group and base, fish group and heat, each on a separate office visit). After completion of the treatments she told me to hold a small portion of fish in my palm and sit for 30 minutes. I felt fine. Then she asked me to eat a small portion of fish. I had my adrenaline near me when I ate a piece of fish, but nothing happened. Ever since I was treated for fish, I eat fish at least twice a week without any problem now. This is the best discovery man (woman) has ever made in medicine.

Dave Moore, L.B., California

Regurgitation

Infants commonly bring up small amounts of milk during or after feeding, especially when burped. Feeding too fast, overfeeding, and swallowing air may cause the infant to regurgitate. Using firm nipples with smaller holes when bottle-feeding should alleviate the problem. However, when the problem continues, the cause may be traced to an allergic reaction to the formula or mother's breast milk.

NAET HELP

Treat for the causative agent if found.
Treat for a sample of the vomit.

Treat NAET group-A, then treat by priority.

Apple cider vinegar 1 drop to 1 ounce of water, and give an ounce every hour until the problem is solved.

ACUHELP: Massage PC-6 for 30 seconds to a minute twice daily and during the attack.

Regurgitation

The parents of a six-month-old boy were concerned because their son was constantly spitting up whenever he was fed. They tried feeding him small amounts very slowly, but he wasn't able to keep his formula down. They changed formula, but he still cried and threw up his formula. Their pediatrician changed the formula to a soy based one to no avail. The infant was still losing weight and crying continuously. We tested him and found that he was allergic to milk, grains, sugars, minerals, soybeans, iron, and corn. Using his mother as a surrogate, he was treated for the basic twelve food groups. After he passed these treatments he was able to drink his formula without crying or spitting up any liquid. His parents came in with a smile on their faces when they came to the clinic with their chubby boy after his first birthday.

Recurrent Abdominal Pain

Three or more episodes of abdominal pains over a three-month period are considered to be recurrent abdominal pain. There are three types of recurrent abdominal pain:

Psychogenic, organic, and functional. Psychogenic recurrent abdominal pain is brought about from stress, anxiety, or depression (recent illness, separation or loss) or at school (concern about grades, teachers, and peers).

Organic recurrent abdominal pain may be due to an organic disorder, most often inflammatory bowel disease, chronic appendicitis, peptic ulcer disease, and urinary tract disease.

Functional recurrent abdominal pain comes from abnormal functioning of an organ. Anxiety may alter autonomic and GI function, causing pain in susceptible persons. All these groups respond well to NAET treatments.

NAET HELP

Treat using NAET for the causative agent if found. Collect a sample of child's saliva at the first sign of the disease and treat with NAET.

If the disease has already progressed, then treat a sample of urine, body secretion, sweat, blood, or stool.

Treat with NAET group-A.

Lemon grass tea or fresh ginger tea 1 ounce as needed.

ACUHELP: Massage all or any of these points for 1-3 minutes: ST-36, LI-4, SP-6 and CV-12.

Supplements

Multizyme 1/2 capsule twice a day.

Fresh ginger tea three times a day.

Agastache formula 1 capsule twice a day.

Abdominal Pains

For three or four months at least twice a week, Darlene would have severe abdominal pain. It became so painful that she would not be able to sleep. She cried and cried through the night. Her frantic mother brought her to see us. We asked her mother what Darlene had been eating for dinner. Her mother said the usual foods she always made. After testing Darlene we found she was reacting to spices. Her mother remembered that about 6 months earlier, she began using spices to flavor her cooking instead of salt, thinking it would be healthier for the family. Darlene was extremely allergic to oregano, rosemary, red chili pepper, and basil. At least twice a week her mother would make Darlene her favorite chicken and pasta. She always used oregano and rosemary on the chicken, and fresh basil and chili pepper on the pasta. After being treated for spices, her abdominal pain stopped.

Allergy to Sugar

Russ, seven-years-old, had severe stomach pains and cramps for three or four months. She took him to the doctor and spent hundreds of dollars for tests, which came back negative. She always tried to keep healthy foods at home to snack on, but lately Russ only wanted sweets. As soon as dinner was finished he would look for a sugary snack. It was just before Christmas when his mother brought Russ to see me. "How long have you had these stomach cramps?" I asked Russ. "Oh, about two months or so," he said. His mother agreed, "They started around the end of October." I tested Russ and found he was allergic to grains and sugars. "Could the pains have started around Halloween? I asked." They both agreed. Ever since Halloween Russ had been craving sweets. It was the first Halloween that Russ' mother had allowed him to go to a Halloween party and then trick or treating with his friends. After the fifth basic treatment (sugar), Russ came in happy as could be. He slept without any stomach cramps for the first night in three months.

Vomiting

Vomiting signals a more serious condition than regurgitation. Repeated projectile vomiting may indicate metabolic disorders, pyloric stenosis, gastroesophageal reflux, small bowel obstruction, and acid-base imbalance. Vomiting with fever and/or lethargy may often mimic an infection (e.g. influenza, viral infection, meningitis). Center for temperature control in the brain is very unstable in young children. Certain allergies to food and drinks can produce severe vomiting and irregular temperature in young children.

NAET HELP

NAET on the causative agent if found.

Treat a sample of vomit from the child each time the child vomits or spits.

Collect a sample of daily food and treat at bed-time.

Treat with NAET group-A, then treat for peptic acid (Stomach acid), sodium bicarbonate, gastric mucosa, collagen, epithelial cells, steroids, alcohol, tobacco smoke, parts of GI tract, DNA/ RNA, bacteria, heliobactor pylori, blood, and immunization drugs, any other drugs taken by the child or the mother during the period of breast feeding or any combinations of the above.

ACUHELP: Massage PC-6 for 30 seconds to a minute during the attack and before eating or drinking.

Supplements

Fresh ginger juice few drops mixed with honey as needed to reduce nausea and vomiting.

Agastache formula one capsule once or twice a day to improve digestive functions.

Apple cider vinegar 1 drop in an ounce of water with sugar or honey to taste, give one ounce every two hours until the nausea subsides.

We would like the parents to learn to test and take care of such acute problems immediately when it occurs. Teachers are the ones with the children during the day. We would like teachers also to learn acute self-help so that when the children fall sick in the school, acute problems can be taken care of immediately before you send them to the hospitals or private doctors.

Projectile Vomiting

6-year-old Mila was brought to our office by her mother at 8:00 a.m. with the complaints of projectile vomiting since 2:00 a.m. without any cause. According to her mother, she had vomited about 12 times by then. She appeared lethargic, had a mild fever, and nauseous. Mila vomited clear yellow liquid once while we were testing her through her mother. Monica, mother of Mila was also our patient getting treated for her migraines. Monica had saved a sample of her vomit from the first batch of vomit in a baby food jar and brought it with her. We immediately treated Mila for the vomit using her mother as surrogate. In less than five minutes Mila was sound asleep. We left her in the room sleeping for an hour. When she awoke, she sat up and said with a smile, "Mom, I am hungry." She was not nauseous anymore.

Vomiting After Meals

A young mother brought an 18-month-old girl to our office because the infant had been vomiting after every meal. She also had severe colicky pains, a skin rash and frequent colds. Testing through NTT, she was found to be allergic to the foods she was eating on a regular basis: chicken, eggs, milk, fruit, salt, and grains. The child was treated through her mother for the basic food groups and her vomiting, colicky pains, and skin rashes disappeared. She gained weight and slept through the night for the first time in her life after clearing the allergy to the grains.

Gastroesophageal Reflux disorder

GER is the regurgitation of the stomach contents into the esophagus, which can cause irritation or inflammation of the esophagus. The disorder is commonly seen in infants. Pain, irritability, inflammation or bleeding of the esophagus, asthma, near-miss SIDS, and pneumonia are associated with GER.

NAET HELP

Treat for the causative agent if found.

Then treat with NAET group-A, then by priority.

ACUHELP: Massage PC-6 for 30 seconds to a minute as needed.

SUPPLEMENTS

Allerplex 1 twice daily.

Agastache formula one capsule twice daily.

Apple cider vinegar 1 drop in an ounce water with sugar or honey to taste, give one ounce every two hours until the nausea subsides.

Allergic to Cereal

A seven-month-old infant began losing weight, vomiting, having difficulties in swallowing. He developed a cough and wheezing. From his symptoms, his pediatrician diagnosed him as having GER. He recommended small, frequent feeding and thickening his cereal. When he was brought to the clinic we traced the problem to the introduction of cereals into his diet. He was allergic to rice, wheat, and corn. After being treated for the basic ten food groups, he began gaining weight, his GER, vomiting, wheezing and cough stopped.

Anorexia

Anorexia Nervosa/Bulimia

Among many eating disorders, anorexia, anorexia nervosa and bulimia are getting much attention nowadays. According to Seattle's Eating Disorders Awareness and Prevention group

(EDAP), an estimated 5-7 percent of America's 12 million undergraduates are afflicted with anorexia (a pathological fear of weight gain leading to extreme weight loss), bulimia (binge and purge syndrome) or binge eating (compulsive overeating). Another recent survey on the weight-obsessed, stressed-out California university coed students showed that 5-10 million females and 1 million males are suffering from eating disorders like anorexia and bulimia. The survey also showed that most of the sufferers are young (from 14 to 25), white, affluent, "perfectionists type-A personalities." According to some of the eating disorder education and prevention groups, the major cause of sudden rise in these disorders is the students' life-style. The college students are away from their families for the first time, and there is tremendous pressure to find their way in the world. Another reason among female victims is due to idolization of wispy models and skinny actresses. A recent UCLA study found that the median recovery time from anorexia is seven years.

According to NAET theory, anorexia, anorexia nervosa and bulimia are a direct result of food allergy. Anorexia is also common in young children. Nausea, vomiting, heartburn, and sour stomach are very frequent symptoms of allergy in the gastrointestinal tract and are usually accompanied by hay fever, asthma, migraine headaches, etc. Energy blockages in the stomach, spleen, liver and heart meridians are usually noted in these cases.

Anorexia nervosa and bulimia (self-induced vomiting after eating) are often also complicated with emotional blockages. In childhood or at a young age, someone may have made a negative remark about the victim's looks, which created an emotional blockage with food and caused the victim to develop bulimia. It could also be due to simple food allergy without any emotional involvement. A qualified NAET practitioner will be able to identify and treat it appropriately.

NAET HELP

Treat using NAET for the causative agent if found.

Treat for the vomit.

NAET group-A.

Then treat for peptic acid (Stomach acid), Sodium bicarbonate, gastric mucosa, collagen, epithelial cells, steroids, alcohol, tobacco smoke, parts of GI tract, DNA/RNA, bacteria, heliobactor pylori, blood, and immunization drugs, any other drugs taken by the child or the mother during the period of breast feeding or any combinations of the above.

Treat a sample of daily food at night before bed time.

ACUHELP: Massage PC-6 and HT-7 for 1-3 minutes every four-six hours through the day as needed.

Supplements

Allerplex 1 twice daily after eliminating the allergies.

Agastache formula one capsule once or twice daily to improve digestive functions.

Betaine HCL 1 pill, with meals.

Multizyme 1 with each meal.

Vitamin C, Vitamin B, vitamin A, trace minerals.

Apple cider vinegar 1 drop in an ounce of water with sugar or honey to taste, give one ounce every two hours until the nausea subsides. This also helps to improve digestion.

Slices of fresh ginger to chew to prevent nausea and vomiting.

Anorexia Nervosa -- A case Study

I suffered from severe anorexia nervosa since I was 17 years old. I felt very fat and ugly especially after I split up with my boy friend. It was a shock to me. I had no desire to eat. My weight dropped to 90 lbs and I am 5'5." Then I met John and he was very different from Sean. He made me realize my problem.

He found out about Dr. Devi and brought me to her for help. My parents, when they found out about my disease, forced me to go for traditional medical treatment. They did not believe in holistic treatments. With my friend's support, I continued with NAET. I felt the difference after 5 NAET treatments. I began taking mega doses of vitamin B complex. That helped to calm my nerves. After 18 treatments, now I can say that I am quite well from my illness. I still have a few more allergies and I am taking care of them slowly. I take a treatment once every three months now. I feel very good and emotionally strong. If it was not for John, Dr. Devi and NAET, I wouldn't be here to tell you my story today.

Susan John, Fullerton, CA

Heartburn

A 8-year-old female child had severe heartburn, sour stomach and frequent vomiting. She happened to be allergic to her own stomach acid secretion. She was treated for her own stomach juice, and that was the end of her heartburn.

Severe intestinal flatulence could be due to poor digestion and absorption of the food in the intestinal tract. It could also be caused by the lack of intestinal enzymes, poor peristaltic movements, too much nitrogen-producing food in the diet (dried beans, etc.) or a symptom of an allergy to the basic or alkaline juice within the intestinal tract.

NAET HELP

Treat using NAET for the causative agent.
Treat for a sample of saliva.
NAET group-A.

Then treat for peptic acid (Stomach acid), Sodium bicarbonate, gastric mucosa, collagen, epithelial cells, steroids, alcohol, tobacco smoke, parts of GI tract, DNA/RNA, bacteria, heliobactor pylori, blood, and immunization drugs, any other drugs taken by the child or the mother during the period of breast feeding or any combinations of the above.

Treat a sample of daily food at night before bed time.

Then treat by priority

ACUHELP: Massage PC-6 and HT-7 for 1-3 minutes every four-six hours through the day.

SUPPLEMENTS

Betaine HCL 1 tab with eah meal.

Multizyme 1 with each meal.

Allergy to Enzymes

Regardless of what type of food he ate, a 44-year-old male would experience severe flatulence and bloating in the abdomen. He was told by a nutritionist not to mix different foods, so he tried eating only one food group at a time. He also took different kinds of enzymes before and after eating, but nothing worked. When he came to us, he was a desperate man. He was relieved of his problems when he was treated for allergy to alkaline juice and digestive enzymes from his intestinal tract.

Since the liver is the first organ that food proteins pass through after entering the blood, it is not surprising to find that allergic manifestations affecting the liver and gall bladder occur with comparative frequency. These manifestations are not necessarily identical; for example, of the two patients having a mild allergy, one patient suffered from enlargement and swelling of the liver while the other patient suffered from intermittent low grade fever. Another patient had his gall bladder removed because of severe abdominal pain. The pain was found to be an allergic reaction to apples and beef. Another man suffered from fainting spells, frequent urination, and mild angina pectoris (heart pains due to an insufficiency of blood supply to the heart muscles), all of these symptoms were relieved by elimination of the offending foods. One patient who suffered from severe upper abdominal pains had her gall bladder removed. Subsequently, she underwent two more abdominal operations only to find out later that the pains were caused by an allergy to eggs and chicken.

Pylorospasm

Pylorospasm, which causes infant colic, is a spasm of the end of the stomach region called the pylorus. The contents of the stomach empty into the intestines through the pylorus. The pylorus is surrounded by folds of mucous membrane containing circular muscular fibers. When an allergy occurs, it causes them to contract spasmodically, similar to the contraction of the bronchial tubes in asthma. This very painful condition causes the child to vomit and cry almost continuously.

NAET HELP

NAET for the causative agent if found.
Treat a sample of child's vomit or saliva.
NAET group-A.
Then treat by priority.
Treat a sample of daily food at night before bed time.
ACUHELP: Massage PC-6 and ST-36 as needed.

Supplements

Allerplex 1 twice daily as needed to reduce the allergic symptoms.

Agastache formula one capsule once or twice daily for children between 2-10 years of age.

Betaine HCL 1 pill, twice daily.

Vitamin C, Vitamin B, vitamin A, and trace minerals.

Apple cider vinegar 1 drop in an ounce of water with sugar or honey to taste, give once every two hours until the nausea subsides.

Pylorospasm and Vomiting

A male child experienced continuous pylorospasm and vomiting after each feeding from the time he was one week old. He also had severe colicky pains, continuous skin rashes, huge hives, ulceration of the gums, heavy tongue coating, thrush, severe diaper rash, frequent colds and high fever, insomnia, and crankiness. He continued to have these symptoms until he was eight months old. His pediatrician suggested minor surgery to tighten the cardiac end or beginning of the stomach, to prevent vomiting. Before he was scheduled for surgery, he was tested by muscle response testing for allergies. The results showed him to be allergic to certain foods. He was treated by NAET soon after. He is a healthy teenager now. He can eat almost any food he wants without any reaction.

Another two-year-old girl with a history of vomiting after each meal was treated in our office. She also had severe colicky pains, continuous skin rashes, huge hives, ulceration of the gums, severe tongue coating, thrush, severe diaper rash, frequent colds and high fever, insomnia, and continuous crying. Her pediatrician prescribed 200 milligrams of Tagamet three times a day. The medication had no effect. She began losing weight and her growth-rate declined. Testing through NTT, she was found to be allergic to all the nutrients and food she was eating. The child was treated in our office for the basic groups (eggs and chicken, milk, vitamin C, fruits, vegetables, B complex vitamins, sugars, iron, vitamin A, salt, minerals and grains). She stopped vomiting after meals, began eating and enjoying food, gained 12 pounds in the three weeks following the treatments, and now she is a beautiful six-year-old healthy girl.

Underfeeding

When infants have been adequately fed they usually fall asleep soon after a feeding. However, if the infant remains restless, cranky, cries and fusses, and awakens 1-2 hours after being fed, he/she may not be getting enough nourishment. If the infant is not gaining weight (>6-8 oz /wk), further investigation may be necessary to determine whether the infant's diet is adequate or appropriate. Underfeeding-like symptom could be an allergy to the food/formula/milk the infant is consuming and the clothes or chemicals on the child (Baby lotion, cream, etc.).

NAET HELP

Treat the child with the daily food sample or any other causative agent if found.

Collect a sample of daily food and treat at bed-time.

Give adequate water between meals.

Talk to the child/infant affectionately (TLC - tender loving care) often, especially after meals.

ACUHELP: Massage St-36 for 1-3 minutes twice daily.

Once I visited my friends (a young couple with a 2 week-old baby) and happened to spend two nights with them. The mother fed the child many times during the night and she said the infant had a huge appetite in the night. The infant still kept crying continuously through the night and the parents were getting upset with the child. Finally they left the child in the bathroom and closed the door. Next morning they told us the story. Every night, if they left the child in the bathroom in a baby carriage (since the baby crib was too large to fit in the small bathroom of their apartment), child slept without crying. Their unique story interested me and I was curious to see if I could trace a cause for this strange problem. My NTT investigation showed that the infant was allergic to the baby crib (Walnut wood). Immediately I treated the infant for the crib, and from that night onwards, baby slept peacefully through the night without crying.

Overfeeding

If the infant gains weight rapidly and regurgitates excessively after meals he/she may be over-fed. Problems with obesity can begin in infancy. However, the symptoms may also be an allergic response to the cereal and formula the infant is being fed, and this can be easily treated with NAET.

NAET HELP

Treat the child with the daily food sample or any other causative agent if found.

Collect a sample of daily food and treat at bed-time.

Treat the spit/vomit immediately as it occurs.

Give adequate water between meals.

Talk to the child/infant affectionately (TLC - tender loving care) often, especially after meals.

ACUHELP: Massage St-36 , PC-6 for 1-3 minutes twice a day and as needed (whenever child is uncomfortable).

Colic

Colic is a disorder which tipically occurs between and 3 and 12 weeks, include episodes of crying and irritability with what appears to be abdominal pain and discomfort. Colic usually begins after the infant is brought home from the hospital and continues until the age of 3 or 4 months. Excessive crying, abdominal pain, and irritability characterize it. The infant may seem excessively hungry and suck vigorously on almost anything. The baby usually turns red and draws his/her legs upward. The excessive crying places undue strain on the family. Colic often occurs at a predictable time, day and night, but some infants cry incessantly. Often the infant's stomach becomes distended and bloated.

A colicky infant may quiet down when held or rocked gently. We have treated infants with colic and most of them have been found to be allergic to the formula and/or liquid they were ingesting. A few drops of apple cider vinegar added in the baby formula or given in water could solve the problem temporarily. Infants with colics are good candidates for future allergic reactions in varying degrees.

NAET HELP

Collect a sample of the baby formula or anything the child ate or drank before the attack and treat the child with emergency Child-help (chapter 9), then treat for NAET group-A.

Acuhelp: Massage ST-36, LI-4 for 30 seconds to a minute as needed.

Supplements

Add a pinch of sodium bicarbonate (baking soda) in a glass of warm water and give one ounce three times a day until the problem solves.

Agastache formula one capsule once or twice daily.

Anise tea 1 teaspoonful before meals.

Ginger tea after meals and at the time of attack.

If your infant sufferers from colic you should find your infant's allergies and eliminate them as soon as possible.

Infant with Colic

I have seen dramatic results on infants with colic. NAET works well on them. When they are on formula or mother's milk, some children get colic. The treatments have very quick and effective results leaving a very happy infant and grateful parents.

Gerald Keyte, D.O., P.C.
Washington, MI.

The parents of a two-month-old girl made an appointment to see me. They hadn't slept a single night since their baby was brought home from the hospital. The baby was restless and it was difficult for her to sleep. She cried constantly, especially after being fed. I noticed she also had a rash on her body and scratch marks. Her parents had tried everything to stop her from crying. They tried giving her a pacifier, creating a quiet environment, using a hot water bottle, and handled her as little as possible, just as the pediatrician told them to do, but nothing stopped the crying. When they telephoned the doctor again to tell him that the baby was screaming more than ever, he said that she should outgrow the colic in a month or two.

Testing the infant with NTT, through the mother as a surrogate, it was found that she was very allergic to her mother's breast milk. The first night after treating for her mother's breast milk, the baby slept through the night without crying. Not only that, on the next visit the baby's parents reported that within 25 hours after the first treatment, the baby's rash and crying disappeared. The baby and her parents sleep through the night now.

Sydney Is Happy, Parents Are Happy!

When sydney as sprawling on the floor at a one year birthday party because she couldn't breathe due to an asthmatic attack due to an allergic reaction, I knew I had to get help. After several trips to the emergency room and advice from our pediatrician, we were able to keep allergy-triggered foods away. However, Sydney couldn't spend the night at anyone's house or even have a playdate.

Any place with pets, dust, goose down bedding etc. was out of the question. Sydney being a very social child, of course wanted to go play at her friends' homes.

Barbara Cesmat introduced me and Sydney to Dr. Devi. Sydney began NAET treatments right away. What a change NAET has made in our lives! Because of NAET, Sydney can play in most homes and can even eat ice cream and cheese pizza. She grew three inches over the past year! She's a soccer goalie! Wow! What a kid!

So this is her advice to other kids: "The best part is the tickling and massage treatment, I love the tickling and massage. The worst part is that you can't eat certain things for a day. But next day you can eat it all!"

"Tell Dr. Devi, thanks for putting a TV in the kids' room."

Thank you Dr. Devi, for giving my daughter a normal life.

Love and many thanks

Beth Fortenberry Tannenbaum

Dear Dr. Abrams,

I am not sure if you will remember me, but I want to thank you anyway. A couple of years ago, I was a patient of yours. I am a dance teacher from Syracuse, and was suffering horribly from food allergies and eczema from head to toe. I was in a really low place in my life, healthwise, and I wanted to update you on my present state of being. I am wonderfully, completely well. I am free of eczema, enjoy wearing sleeveless shirts, shorts, and bare feet for the first time in years. My energy level is amazing, now that all of my energy is not going into constantly trying to heal. I met a wonderful man and got married, and we are expecting a baby boy in January of 2001. I want you to know how deeply you touched my life and what a difference you and NAET made in the quality of life that I now am able to enjoy.

Susan Hughes, New York

NAET Practitioner:
Judy Abrams, L.Ac
Ithaca, NY

CHAPTER 6

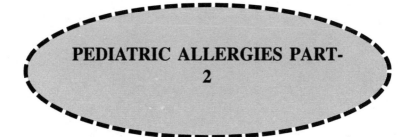

PEDIATRIC ALLERGIES PART-2

6

PEDIATRIC ALLERGIES
PART-2

INFLAMMATORY BOWEL DISEASES

The root cause of most of the diseases often found in the gut beginning with nausea, poor digestion, heartburn, reflux, bloating, cramps, diarrhea, gas, constipation, abdominal pains, nervous stomach, etc. is allergy. If not taken care of immediately, they can lead to cough, colds and flu, fever, sinusitis, bronchitis, heart attacks, migraines, mental and emotional imbalances, irritabilities, arthritis, Crohn's disease, ulcerative colitis, irritable bowel syndrome, bladder infection, menstrual disorders, skin disorders, stroke, cancer and even death.

Inflammatory bowel diseases are chronic inflammatory diseases of the gastrointestinal tract. Based on clinical, endoscopic and histological findings, inflammatory bowel diseases are categorized into two groups: Ulcerative colitis and Crohn's disease.

The inflammatory response in ulcerative colitis is largely confined to the colon and affects mucosa and submucosa whereas Crohn's disease can involve any part of the gastrointestinal tract, and the inflammation can extend through the intestinal wall from mucosa to serosa.

According to one of the latest report from CDC, the highest affected people are white races in northern Europe and north America, at a prevalence rate of about 50 per 100,000. Rates are higher in upper income groups than lower income groups. The peak age at onset is between 15 and 25. Approximately 15% of IBD patients have an affected first-degree relative. The incidence is equal in men and women. The incidence is increasing over the last forty years, for undetermined reasons. Environmental factors can act on the genetic background of an individual to influence expression of the disease.

Common Symptoms to both diseases:

Diarrhea usually associated with blood; slow onset but insidious; frequent small volume stool with urgency and occasional incontinence; lower quadrant rectal pain; fever, malaise; weight loss.

Usually follows a chronic, relapsing and remitting course, with attacks lasting for days to weeks or even months at a time.

NAET HELP

Collect a sample of the stool in a test tube and treat the child with NAET.

Find the causative agent for the present attack and treat for the allergen using NAET or avoid the allergen.

Treat for NAET group-A, then treat by priority.
Treat the sample of urine, body secretion, sweat, stool, venous blood, bacteria, virus and parasite.
Avoid raw and uncooked food.
ACUHELP: ST-36, SP-6, SP-10, ST-40, and LI-11.

Supplements

Vitamin C, Vitamin B, vitamin A, trace minerals. Allerplex 1 twice daily as needed to reduce the allergic symptoms.
Calcium lactate 1 pill three times daily.
Agastache formula one capsule once or twice daily.
Arrowroot or rice water 1/2 cup at the start of the meal.
Overcook the vegetables and grains before feeding. Overcooking will help the nutrients to absorb faster and they do not cause irritation of the gastrointestinal tract.

Through NTT, our patients with IBD have been found to be highly allergic to foods and bacteria. When they get treated for most of their food allergies, and bacteria mix they become free of symptoms and pain.

Irritable Bowel Syndrome

Irritable bowel syndrome (IBS) is a disorder effecting the intestines. According to western medical researchers, no particular cause has been found; however, diet, drugs, hormones and emotional factors have been found as major triggers.

The commonly experienced symptom of IBS is pain in the abdomen, predominantly after meals. Other symptoms are periodic diarrhea or constipation, lower abdominal pain, pain after eating, bowel movements immediately after eating, cramps in the lower abdomen, bloating, flatulence, nausea, headache, depression, fatigue, anxiety and poor concentration.

NAET HELP

Treat for the causative agent if the child has an acute attack. Collect a sample of the stool in a test tube and treat the child with NAET.

Find the causative agent and treat if possible or avoid the allergen.

Then treat with classic NAET groups by priority..

Eat allergy-free, very well cooked vegetables, fruits and food.

ACUHELP: Massage ST-36, SP-4, SP-10 and LI-11.

Supplements

Allerplex 1 twice daily as needed to reduce the allergic symptoms.

Calcium lactate 1 pill three times daily.

Agastache formula one capsule once or twice daily for children between 2-10 years of age.

Arrowroot or rice water 1/2 cup at the start of the meal.

Overcook the vegetables and grains before feeding. Overcooking will help the nutrients to absorb faster and they do not cause irritation of the gastrointestinal tract.

Through NTT, our patients with IBS have been found to be highly allergic to foods. When they get treated for most of their food allergies, they become free of symptom and pain.

Colitis

This is characterized by looseness of bowels, diarrhea, colic, belching, vomiting and varying symptoms of the stomach and intestines. Very often allergic in origin, certain types of colitis are caused by amoeba (parasite) and bacteria. This type of colitis or dysentery is very common in the tropics, and parasites are frequently brought into the country by returning travelers. In these cases, most of the time the parasites are allergens. However, the parasitical type of colitis is usually quite readily diagnosed by laboratory methods. When these tests are negative, it is wise to consider the possibility of allergy. Another type of colitis, called nonspecific colitis, cannot be diagnosed by laboratory tests. This type usually occurs in nervous, excitable or unstable individuals with the nervous state being blamed for the colitis. Extremely nervous individuals may be allergic to their own adrenaline. Extreme nervousness often accompanies and aggravates various allergic manifestations, such as colitis. These people are also very allergic to B complex vitamins.

Allergies to milk, wheat, grains, gluten, spices, and fruits are the most frequent causes of allergic colitis. To a lesser degree, allergies to vegetables, fish, meat, and other foods will also undoubtedly be responsible for this condition.

NAET HELP

Collect a sample of the stool in a test tube and treat the child with NAET.

Find the causative agent and treat if possible or avoid the allergen.

Then treat with classic NAET groups by priority. groups.

Eat very well cooked vegetables and food. Avoid raw and uncooked food.

ACUHELP: SP-4, SP-10 and LI-4.

Supplements

Allerplex 1 twice daily as needed to reduce the allergic symptoms.

Calcium lactate 1 pill three times daily.

Agastache formula one capsule twice daily.

Betaine HCL 1 pill, twice daily with meals.

Multizyme 1 capsule twice a day with meals.

Celiac Disease

Celiac disease is characterized by a permanent intolerance to gluten, which leads to changes of the small intestine. Gluten is a complex molecule found in wheat, rye, oats, and barley. The most common age for children to be diagnosed with celiac disease is between one and five years of age. Diarrhea, vomiting, loss of appetite, delayed onset of puberty, dyspepsia (difficulty swallowing), arthritis and joint pain, mental retardation, and neurological problems are symptoms of celiac disease. NAET treatments are very effective in treating this disease. Allergies to every day foods such as wheat, grains, milk, spices, fats, beans, and meat, can cause the symptoms of celiac disease.

Mucous colitis

Mucous colitis, has very similar symptoms to those of ordinary colitis, except that large quantities of mucus are formed in the intestine and passed through the bowels. At one time this condition was known as "asthma of the bowels," which frequently occurs in people who have other allergic manifestations like asthma. The respiratory tract and the intestines are lined with the same kind of mucous membranes. Large quantities of mucus form in the respiratory tract when a person has bronchial asthma, and the same thing happens in the intestines when an allergy affects the bowels.

NAET HELP

Treat for the causative agent if found.

Collect a sample of child's stool at the first sign of the disease and treat with NAET.

Then treat with NAET group-A.

Eat very-well-cooked vegetables and food. Avoid raw and uncooked food.

ACUHELP: SP-4, SP-10 and LI-4.

Supplements

Vitamin C, Vitamin B, vitamin A, Trace minerals, allerplex 1 twice daily as needed to reduce the allergic symptoms.
Agastache formula one capsule once or twice daily.
Betaine HCL 1 pill, twice daily.
Apple cider vinegar 1 drop in an ounce of water with sugar or honey to taste, give one ounce every two hours as needed.

Diarrhea

Diarrhea is one of the most significant medical problems throughout the world. In the USA alone there are between 20-40 million episodes of diarrhea in children less than five-years-old. About 200,000 children are hospitalized in the USA with severe diarrhea and 200-400 die each year.

Acute Diarrhea

Acute diarrhea is the Sudden onset of frequent loose, watery stools, or unformed bowel movements. The colon, small intestines, rectum, and skin around the rectum are involved.

Signs And Symptoms

Abdominal pain with cramps.
Loose, watery or unformed bowel movements.
Lack of bowel control
Fever (sometimes).

Possible Causes

Food Allergy
Food Poisoning.
Viral, bacteria or parasitic infections.
Disease or tumor of the pancreas.
Consuming excessive amount of high fiber food like prunes.

NAET HELP

Treat for the causative agent if found.

Collect a sample of child's stool and treat.

Treat NAET group-A, then treat by priority.

If cramps are present, place mild heat compresses on the abdomen.

If it is food poisoning, give activated charcoal, 1 pill immediately and repeat once after two hours.

Apple cider vinegar 1 drop in 1 ounce water (add sugar to taste), give an ounce every hour by mouth. You may also give the child ginger tea, green tea, ginger ale, etc. This will hydrate the child, add enough acid to the stomach and helps to digest the undigested food, improve elimination and reduce nausea.

If the child is bloated or has flatulence, give anise tea 1 ounce after meals.

Blend an over-ripe banana in buttermilk, add sugar to taste and feed one ounce every two hours.

If the child has profuse diarrhea, appears severely dehydrated, the child may need hospitalization.

After the acute phase, take the child to an NAET practitioner and get the NAET basics treated.

ACUHELP: St-36, Sp-4, LI-4, SP-10.

Chronic Diarrhea

Loose bowel movements that may occur in infants and children are normally no cause for alarm unless accompanied by weight loss, passage of blood, and/or failure to gain weight. But in chronic diarrhea a healthy child may have more than 5 watery stools a day.

A low-grade diarrhea persisting for weeks or months.

• An infection causing diarrhea with vomiting, bloody stools, fever, or listlessness.

• An on-going allergy to every day food or drinks.

• Sugar malabsorption, gluten allergy and allergic gastroenteritis. Intolerance to milk protein, carbohydrate, lactose or glucose. It is often present in infancy and childhood and is frequently associated with colic, eczema, and vomiting. When the child grows up, the diarrhea may subside, but the allergy may be manifested in other symptoms. There are cases in which diarrhea continues throughout adulthood if the allergy is not identified and treated.

NAET HELP

Collect a sample of child's stool and treat daily.

Treat for classic NAET groups.

If cramps are present, place mild heat compresses on the abdomen.

Apple cider vinegar 1 drop in 1 ounces water (add sugar to taste), give an ounce every hour by mouth.

Ginger tea, green tea, ginger ale, etc., as needed.

If the child is bloated or has flatulence, give anise tea 1 ounce after meals.

Blend an over-ripe banana in buttermilk, add sugar to taste and feed one ounce two times a day.

ACUHELP: ST-36, SP-4, SP-10.

Supplements

Agastache formula one capsule once or twice daily for children between 2-10 years of age.

Betaine HCL 1 pill, twice daily.

Multizyme 1 twice daily.

According to oriental medical principle, weak spleen meridian causes diarrhea. Spleen weakness also causes bleeding disorders. Patients with intestinal allergies also have a tendency to bleed from various parts of their body. Don's mother couldn't remember when he didn't have nosebleeds and bloodshot eyes (conjunctiva) along with diarrhea. Checking Don, we found that the milk he was drinking everyday was the cause of his problems. After he passed the milk/calcium treatment, not only did his diarrhea stop, but his nosebleeds and bloodshot eyes also disappeared.

Constipation

Constipation means difficult or uncomfortable bowel movements. A combination of changes in the frequency, size, and ease of stool passage may be seen leading to a decrease in bowel movements. The colon and the entire intestinal tract are involved.

Any of the following may be a sign of constipation.

• The opposite condition of diarrhea, it can also be a symptom of an allergy. Infrequent bowel movements, sometimes accompanied by abdominal swelling, and bloating.

• Hard feces.

• Straining during bowel movements

• Pain or bleeding with bowel movements.

Sensation of continuing fullness after a bowel movement.

Possible causes

• Inadequate fluid intake.

• Insufficient fiber in the diet. Fiber adds bulk, holds water, and creates easy passage for the stool.

• Inactivity.

• Hypothyroidism.

• Hypercalcemia.

• Anal fissure.

• Depression.

• Chronic kidney failure.

• Backaches.

• Spasms of the small bowel due to food allergy.

The smooth muscle of the colon is a logical site for allergic spasm and could easily cause this condition. The intestines are lined with mucous membrane, so it is possible for large quantities of mucus to form in them, just as it does in nasal passages. In severe allergic constipation, the muscle of the colon may contract to such a degree that very little food passes through the channel in a normal manner.

NAET HELP

Collect a sample of the baby formula or food in a test tube and treat the child with NAET.

NAET group-A.

Soak raisins overnight and cook it in the morning, blend it well and feed one ounce of pureed raisins twice a day.

Make the child drink adequate amount of water.

ACUHELP: ST-37 bilateral.

Supplements

Agastache formula one capsule once or twice daily.

Betaine HCL 1 pill, twice daily.

Multizyme 1 cap. twice daily.

Teach your child normal bowel habits. Set aside a regular time each day for your child's bowel movements. The best time is often within 1 hour after breakfast, lunch and dinner. A normal person should move his/her bowel once after major meals.

• Encourage the child to drink adequate amount of clear water or lemonade. Divide your child's body weight in pounds by two and give him/her that many ounces of water daily. A child weighing 40 pounds, should drink 20 ounces of water daily spaced through the day.

• Mix apple cider vinegar 1 teaspoonful in 8 ounces of water and give 1 ounce after each meal and pancreatic lipase 100 mgs 30 minutes after each meal.

• Prune juice 1 ounce every night after supper might help.

Make sure your child gets enough exercise daily.

About a teaspoonfull of honey added to an ounce of warm prune juice, followed with a cup of other warm drink might help to relieve severe acute constipation in children. When the acute situation clears up, you must find the cause of the constipation and eliminate the problem.

Constipation

Tina, 4-years-old, had been suffering from long bouts of constipation. Her mother tried everything from bran cereal, bulk fruits, vegetables, and fibers to help alleviate the condition but nothing seemed to work. Tina's stomach was so bloated she could only wear pants with elastic waistbands. Testing through NTT we found that Tina was not only severely allergic to the raw carrots her mother was giving her as a snack everyday, but also allergic to all the fibers she was eating to eliminate the constipation! Now that she has been treated for the NAET group-A food groups, she fits into her pants and wears a belt comfortably. Best of all her painful constipation is gone.

Drugs Taken by the Mother

Drugs taken by the mother during breast-feeding may cause mild to severe reactions in the infant depending on the type of drug, the dosage taken, and its half-life. Drugs that are not usually hazardous to the infant include insulin and epinephrine, which do not pass into breast milk.

My Child Was Allergic to Anesthesia!!

My twenty-month-old daughter Olivia has never stood or walked alone. At six months of age, she had surgery on both feet for a condition known as Vertical Talus. Her feet healed nicely and on schedule from the operation.

Upon a check up visit to the surgeon, I expressed my concern that my daughter wasn't standing alone or walking. The doctor examined her and told me he didn't see a physical reason for this delay and referred her to a neurologist who would test her nerve endings.

Having been familiar with NAET for a couple of years, I took Olivia to Dr. Prince for treatment. After hearing of her surgery which required anesthesia, Olivia was tested and found allergic to anesthesia. She was treated for this on Friday afternoon. That night Olivia stood alone for the first time. Two days later she was walking alone.

My husband and I are convinced the allergy to anesthesia was the reason for Olivia's delayed walking skills. We're so grateful to Dr. Devi Nambudripad for developing this technique and sharing it with the world.

Karen Hyatt
Monroe, North Carolina

Caffeine is not well excreted by the infant and may accumulate, causing irritability and allergic reactions. Some children are very sensitive to the smell of the coffee brewing. If a small child develops irritability, sinusitis, runny nose, itchy skin or asthma in the morning hours while their parents are busy brewing coffee in the house, it is the smell of the coffee.

Coffee Smell Triggered Asthma

Three months ago four-year-old Tanya began treatment with us for her severe asthmatic disorder that started from the time she was brought home on her third day of her life. She was on two inhalers and cortisone. The asthma medication helped to reduce the intensity of attacks but they were never eliminated completely. According to her mother her lungs never ever stopped

wheezing completely. Her mother was very particular in follow-
ing directions. Tanya completed NAET group-A. She still woke
up with asthma. Her asthma improved as the day progressed.
She even began sleeping better through the night without short-
ness of breath or asthma. But waking up with asthma still puzzled
everyone.

Then we chose to treat her for chocolate since one of her
questions lately was: "can she eat chocolate cake for her birth-
day."

Chocolate treatment also required them to refrain from
coffee and coffee brewing smell. So her father couldn't brew
coffee in the house. That was the first morning she woke up with-
out any breathing difficulties. After her successful treatment for
coffee, chocolate and caffeine, Tanya's morning asthma said
good-bye to her. She hasn't had any asthma for three years now.

Alcohol intake should be limited and mothers should not
breast-feed within two hours of smoking. Drugs that suppress or
inhibit lactation include estradiol, large-dose contraceptives,
levodopa, and the antidepressant trazodone. Almost all antibiotics
are usually excreted in milk; infants may develop hypersensitivity,
diarrhea, or candidiasis. Tetracycline and penicillin are excreted
in breast milk. Any drug excreted in breast milk can cause an
allergic reaction in an infant.

Allergy to Cocaine

Angela had lived with her grandmother since she was an
infant. It was difficult for Angela's grandmother but she loved
her granddaughter very much and was managing very well
until Angela started school. By first grade she was placed in a
learning disability class. She was hyperactive, had a short attention span, did not do class work or read any words. The
teacher called Angela's grandmother to inform her that her

behavior with the other children was getting out of hand. She pushed, threw things, yelled, and hit anyone near her. The teacher didn't think Angela would be able to continue in a regular class setting. When Angela's grandmother brought her to the clinic she was uncontrollable, running up and down the hall, screaming at her grandmother. We tested her and found that she was allergic to everything she was eating. When her grandmother told us that Angela's mother had taken drugs before Angela was born, we tested her for cocaine and marijuana. She was highly allergic to them. We started her on the basic treatments immediately. As she passed each treatment her hyperactivity and disruptive behavior was reduced. After the basic ten treatments Angela's grandmother met with her teacher. The teacher was amazed she couldn't believe the change in Angela. She began reading and counting. She rarely hit or yelled and she would be able to stay in a regular first grade class. After she was treated for marijuana and cocaine Angela did not need to receive special reading instructions. She is now in the third grade and reading fifth grade books. She has been on the honor roll at her school. Her grandmother is as proud as she can be.

Smoking/Nicotine

Secondary smoke is a major problem to the children when their relatives smoke around them. Children who are sensitive to cigarette or tobacco smoke suffer from upper respiratory disorders like frequent asthma, bronchitis, pneumonia, sinusitis, shortness of breath, brain irritation, poor concentration, poor growth and development, autoimmune disorders, cancer, etc. In the U.S. cigarette smoking is reduced in the past year. Smoking is not allowed in the public places, public eating places, offices, etc. But it is a major problem in the developing countries and third world countries and in other countries like in Europe.

NAET HELP

NAET treatments on cigarette and smoke will help your child to handle the immediate allergic reactions resulting from smoke. Please check with your practitioner for more information on treating your child's allergy to cigarette and nicotine. After completing the treatment, you should avoid the exposure to smoke for your child to maintain the health achieved by treating the allergy to smoke.

Eczema

Eczema (dermatitis) is one of the most irritating and distressing skin conditions which could have profound effects on a sufferer's health, happiness and life-style. As many as one in ten children may be affected at some time in their childhood. This is an inflammation of the upper layers of the skin, causing blisters, redness, swelling, oozing, scabbing, scaling and itching. Continuous scratching and rubbing may eventually lead to thickening and hardening of the skin. These can often weep, leading to crusting and scabs, leaving patches of raw skin. The skin itches constantly and may be painful. Skin lesions can get infected at times. Scratching can also cause bleeding and secondary infection.

NAET HELP

If it is an acute case, using NTT testing procedures find the causative agent if possible and give emergency NAET on your child.

Treat for NAET group-A, then treat by priority.

Then Collect a sample of the baby formula or any other food the child is eating in a test tube and treat the child with NAET.

At home, collect samples of foods from daily meals and treat daily at bedtime.

Hibiscus tea 1/2 cup twice a day.

Apply milk of magnesia or calamine lotion locally to prevent itching.

ACUHELP: LI-11, SP-10, PC-6.

Supplements

Agastache formula one capsule once or twice daily for children between 2-10 years of age.

Betaine HCL 1 pill, twice daily.

Multizyme 1 daily

Allerplex 1 cap once or twice daily as needed.

Antioxidant 1 daily.

Essential fatty acids 1 daily

Adequate water intake

If the bowels are not moving once or twice a day, mild herbal laxatives can be used.

Epsom salt bath once or twice a day to reduce itching and swelling if there is any. (Add a cup of Epsom salt to the lukewarm water in bath tub and make the child soak in the water for 30 minutes at a time. Please check for allergies of the products before you use.

Contact Dermatitis

This is an inflammation caused by contact with a particular substance; the rashes confined to a specific area and often has clearly defined boundaries. Common causes of contact dermatitis include irritation and/or allergic reaction from the following:

• Cosmetics: shampoo, conditioner, hair-removing chemicals, nail polish, nail polish remover, deodorants, moisturizers, after-shave lotions, perfumes, sunscreens, eye makeup, skin lotions and creams of various kinds, lipstick, and lip gloss.

• Chemicals used in clothing manufacturing: tanning agents in shoes, rubber products, latex products, plastic products, shoes, undergarments, chemicals in commonly used other fabrics, dry cleaning chemicals, fabric or covering of sofa, chair, hand bag, shoulder bags, wood or other materials on a writing desk, computer or typewriter keyboard, plastic or wooden pens or pencils, head bands and clips.

• Metal compounds: Different types of jewelry, wedding ring (worn continuously on the finger), copper, silver, nickel, gold, stainless steel, metal chairs, and tools used frequently for work or hobby.

• Drugs in skin creams: antibiotics, antihistamines, anesthetics, antiseptics, and stabilizers.

• Plants: Poison ivy, poison oak, poison sumac, trees, wood work, ragweed, grasses, flowers, house plants, and plants in the garden if contacting them.

• Materials: Animals and their products: goose down, animal fur, animal saliva, and hair, fibers of bed linens (for example: cotton, polyester, acrylic, wool, nylon, feather), pillows, pillow cases, clothes, socks, hats, elastic, stuffed animals, books, paper, toilet paper, hand towels, cellular phone, and the list can go on.

NAET HELP

If it is an acute case, using NTT testing procedures find the causative agent if possible and give emergency NAET on your child.

Treat for NAET group-A, then treat by priority.

Then Collect a sample of the baby formula or any other food the child is eating in a test tube and treat the child with NAET.

At home, collect samples of foods from daily diet and treat every night before bedtime.

ACUHELP: LI-11, SP-10

Supplements

Agastache formula one capsule once or twice daily for children between 2-10 years of age.
Betaine HCL 1 pill, twice daily.
Multizyme 1 daily
Allerplex 1 cap once or twice daily as needed.
Antioxidant 1 daily.
Essential fatty acids 1 daily
Adequate water intake
Herbal Laxatives if necessary
Milk of magnesia or calamine lotion locally to reduce itching.

Epsom salt bath once or twice a day to reduce itching and swelling if there is any. Add a cup of Epsom salt to the lukewarm water in bath tub and make the child soak in the water for 30 minutes at a time. Please check for allergies of the products before you use as always.

Fourteen year Itch!

For 14 years I suffered from an itch around the left side of my waist line, which caused my skin to turn dark brown. I was tested for skin cancer, treated for candida, yeast, and went through cleansing programs of various kinds over the years with no results. My itching began spreading into my thighs instead of getting better. Finally I discovered Dr. Devi. In her office she tested me for elastic and found that it was the cause of my problem. Since I was not allergic to very many foods, she treated me for the elastics on my first visit. What relief I got from that one treatment! My waistline never itched again!

Pam Bain, El Segundo, CA

The effects of contact dermatitis range from a mild, short-lived redness to severe swelling and blisters. Often the rash contains tiny, itching blisters. At first, the rash is limited to the contact site, but later it may spread. The rash area may be very small (for example: ear lobes if earrings cause dermatitis), or it may cover a large area of the body (for example: if a body lotion causes dermatitis).

Diaper Rash

My son was five days old when Doctor Devi began to treat him for cotton so he could wear his diapers. When my baby returned for the next treatment, it was for a terrible diaper rash, because he had a reaction to my breast milk. Dr. Devi traced this to the peanut butter I had eaten. Bill, my baby boy, had thrown up and had diarrhea all night long. His bottom, as a result was "raw" by morning. After Dr. Devi treated the baby and me for the allergy to peanut butter, the rash and rawness disappeared completely in exactly 24 hours.

Debbie White, La Habra, CA

Determining the cause of contact dermatitis isn't always easy because the possibilities of contacts are endless. Also, people aren't aware of all the substances that touch the skin. Often the location of the initial rash is an important clue.

Allergy to Cotton

A one-month-old baby was brought into the clinic with an oozing rash all over her body. The mother had been using an ointment on the infant that her pediatrician gave her for two weeks but the rash was getting worse. We tested the baby through her mother (as a surrogate) and found that she was allergic to the clothing, diapers, and blankets she was in contact with. They all were made from cotton. After treating her for cotton her severe case of contact dermatitis disappeared.

Traditional testing procedure are cumbersome and/or painful and may not provide the expected results often. A patch test is complicated since the possibilities of allergens are endless. If at all possible your doctor might do patch tests on one or two allergens at a time; it can take years before one completes the testing alone. Even though time consuming, NTT offers a better solution in the diagnostic area since many items can be tested painlessly and more accurately. The main traditional treatment for dermatitis is avoidance of the substance other than taking cortisone, or antiinflammatory drugs or symptomatic drugs. NAET is the only treatment that can eliminate the allergies to contacted items painlessly and give the sufferer quick relief.

Chronic Dermatitis

This includes a group of disorders in which a particular part of the body, usually an area around the mouth, buttocks, hip area, hands and feet are frequently inflamed and irritated. Chronic dermatitis of these areas results from repetitive exposures and contacts with the chemicals, or materials. For example: allergy to diaper, pacifier, feeding bottles, rubber nipples, the (latex) rubber lined training pants, tethers, toys, washing soaps, bath tub toys, baby seats, hand towels, shoes and socks. Chronic dermatitis may make the skin of the affected area itch or hurt. It can also produce itchy blisters and oozing or bleeding from the site due to scratching.

If you pay enough attention, this type of condition is easier to trace than that of contact dermatitis. This often overlaps contact dermatitis. In contact dermatitis the lesion may stay mostly at the site of contact or may spread all over the body. In chronic dermatitis, lesion may affect the area of contact only. NAET can eliminate the allergies to contacted items painlessly and give the sufferer quick relief.

NAET HELP

Treat for NAET group-A, then treat by priority.

Then Collect a sample of the baby formula or any other food the child is eating in a test tube and treat the child with NAET.

At home, collect samples of foods and treat before bedtime.

ACUHELP: LI-11, SP-10, PC-6.

Supplements

Agastache formula one capsule once or twice daily.

Betaine HCL 1 pill, twice daily.

Multizyme 1 daily.

Allerplex 1 cap once or twice daily as needed.

Essential fatty acids 1 daily.

Adequate water intake.

Herbal laxative as needed. Milk of magnesia locally to reduce itching.

Epsom salt bath once or twice a day to reduce itching and swelling if there is any. Add a cup of Epsom salt to the lukewarm water in bath tub and make the child soak in the water for 30 minutes at a time.

The Stubborn Eczema

Tanya was four months old when she began to have eczema that covered her body. Her skin would crack, bleed and get infected. We noticed it would get worse and the itching progressed when we were out of doors. Doctors gave us many creams to try and we got no results from them. We heard of NAET from a friend and gave it a try. It was really amazing to see her get treated for environmental things such as sunlight, heat, grass, etc. Her skin slowly healed and only a small spot on her thumb bothers her sometimes versus her entire body.

Tanya Wilber, North Carolina

Atopic Dermatitis

This is a chronic, itchy inflammation of the upper layers of the skin that often develops in people who have history of other hypersensitivity reactions in themselves or in their family members. People with atopic dermatitis usually have many other allergic disorders. Some people may have an inherited tendency to produce excessive antibodies, such as immunoglobulin E in response to a number of different stimuli. Many conditions can make atopic dermatitis worse, including emotional stress, changes in temperature, humidity, bacterial skin infections, contact with irritating clothing, different kinds of food, and many environmental factors.

Atopic dermatitis sometimes appears in the first few months after birth. Infants may develop red, oozing, crusted rashes on the face, scalp, diaper area, hands, arms, feet, or legs. Often the dermatitis clears up by age 3 or 4, although it commonly recurs. In older children the rash often occurs or recurs in only one or two spots, especially on the upper arms, in front of the elbows or behind the knees.

NAET HELP

Treat for NAET group-A, then treat by priority.

Collect a sample of the baby formula or any other food the child is eating in a test tube and treat the child with NAET.

At home, collect samples of foods from daily diet and treat before bedtime.

ACUHELP: LI-11, SP-10, PC-6.

Supplements

Agastache formula one capsule once or twice daily for children between 2-10 years of age.

Betaine HCL 1 pill, twice daily.

Multizyme 1 daily

Allerplex 1 cap once or twice daily as needed.

Epsom salt bath once or twice a day to reduce itching and swelling if there is any. Add a cup of Epsom salt to the lukewarm water in bath tub and make the child soak in the water for 30 minutes at a time.

Seborrheic Dermatitis

This is an inflammation of the upper layers of the skin, causing scales on the scalp, face, and occasionally on other areas. Seborrheic dermatitis often run in families, and cold weather usually makes it worse.

Seborrheic dermatitis usually begins gradually, causing dry, greasy scaling of the scalp (dandruff), sometimes with itching but without hair loss. In more severe cases, yellowish to reddish scaly pimples appear along the hairline, behind the ears, in the ear canal, on the eyebrows, on the bridge of the nose, around the nose, and on the chest. In newborns less than a month old, seborrheic dermatitis may produce a thick, yellow, crusted scalp rash (cradle cap) and sometimes yellow scaling behind the ears and red rashes on the face. Frequently diaper rash accompanies the scalp rash. Older children may develop a thick, tenacious, scaly rash with large flakes of skin.

Milk, mother's milk, milk products, baby shampoo, soap, baby oils, fats in the food, egg products in the food, skin lotions, etc. have been found to be the causative agents by testing through NTT. Treatments with NAET often gives quicker and lasting results.

NAET HELP

Treat for NAET group-A, then treat by priority. Then Collect a sample of the baby formula or any other food the child is eating in a test tube and treat the child with NAET. Collect samples of foods taken during the day and treat using child-help points before bedtime.
ACUHELP: LI-11, SP-10, PC-6.

Supplements

Agastache formula one capsule once or twice daily for children between 2-10 years of age.

Betaine HCL 1 pill, twice daily.

Allerplex 1 cap once or twice daily as needed.

Antioxidant 1 daily.

Essential fatty acid 1 daily.

Milk of magnesia can be applied locally to reduce itching.

Wash the head with Vinegar bath once every other day to reduce itching and swelling if there is any. Add 1 cup vinegar to three gallons of lukewarm water. Protect the child's eyes.

Olive oil can be applied on the skin prevent dryness.

Apply hibiscus-leaf paste on the head and leave it for 30 minutes. Then wash the head with olive leaf or lemon leaf bath. Hibiscus-leaf-paste can be used instead of shampoo. (Grind up fresh hibiscus leaves to a fine paste and use the paste to wash the head or other areas with eczema or dermatitis).

You may continue all other medications you are using on child while you follow these treatments. There are no contraindications with NAET if you want to give any other treatments or products while the child is receiving NAET as long as you check for allergy to the products.

Acne

Acne begins at puberty. Since our generation of children are reaching puberty earlier than their pioneer counterparts (many of our young children have reached puberty by the age of ten), acne begins at a young age to some of them. Acne is a common inflammatory pilosebaceous diesease characterized by papules, pustules, inflamed nodules, superficial pus-filled cysts, and in extreme cases, deep, inflamed, purulent sacs. From NAET point of view, acne is caused by an interaction between hormones, sebum, sweat, bacteria, vitamin C, B complex, sugar, iron, vitamin A, salt, minerals, corn, grains, spices, fats, deep fried foods, and combination of any of these.

NAET HELP

If it is an acute case, find the causative agent if possible and give emergency NAET on your child.

Treat NAET group-A, then treat by priority.

Then Collect samples of the daily foods in a test tube and treat the child with NAET.

At home, collect samples of foods taken during the day and treat using self-help points before bedtime.

ACUHELP: LI-11, SP-10, PC-6.

Supplements

Persica and Rhubarb formula one capsule once or twice daily

Betaine HCL 1 pill, twice daily.

Allerplex 1 cap once or twice daily as needed.

Essential fatty acid 1 daily.

Milk of magnesia can be applied locally to reduce itching.

Wash the face or affected area with Vinegar bath once or twice a day to reduce itching and swelling if there is any. Add 1 cup vinegar to three gallons of water. Protect the child's eyes.

Bacterial Infections

Diphtheria

Diphtheria is an acute contagious disease spread chiefly by the secretions of infected persons. The organisms ordinarily lodge in the tonsils or nasopharynx. As they multiply they produce lethal toxins carried by the blood, which damage cells in organs and create lesions in respiratory passages, the nervous system, and the kidneys. Initially, the patient has a mild sore throat, a low-grade fever, increased heart rate, and rising leukocytosis. In children, nausea, fever and chills are common. Active immunization with DPT vaccine is routinely given in this country. The DPT antitoxin (which is derived from horses), can also cause a reaction. Children can be allergic to the DPT vaccine itself causing several allergic reactions including symptoms such as learning disabilities, hyperactivity, and allergic autism.

NAET HELP

Children can be tested by NTT to see if they would react to the vaccine before being inoculated. If the child is found to be allergic to the vaccine, he/she should be treated using NAET before being inoculated.

If the child is manifesting acute symptoms within hours of injection, provide acute NAET care using a fresh sample of vaccine, or any of the body secretions if the vaccine is not available: saliva, urine, vomit or blood.

If the child is having after-effects of vaccination, follow the classic NAET protocol for basic treatments with a practitioner.

Then collect samples of the daily foods in a test tube and treat the child with NAET.

Treat DPT vaccine and all combinations with NAET
ACUHELP: LI-11, SP-10, PC-6 and Kid-6.

Supplements

Calcium lactate 1 pill (standard process lab of so. Ca.) four times a day.

B vitamins 100 mgs daily in devided doses.

Betaine HCL 1 pill, twice daily.

Multizyme 1 capsule twice a day after meals.

Allerplex 1 cap once or twice daily as needed.

Essential fatty acid 1 daily.

Multivitamin as needed.

Allergic to DPT Vaccination

Two weeks after Ricky received his DPT vaccine he was running a high fever (103-104 degrees), had flu symptoms and became very moody. He was given Tylenol and later antibiotics. After almost a month his fever and flu symptoms stopped, but his parents noticed a change in him. His attention span was different. He couldn't sit still for a moment. He was always moving around. He didn't even listen to his mother when she read him his favorite story. The most unnerving part was that he forgot what he had learned. Prior to DPT he loved counting to ten and saying the alphabet. Everyone considered him to be a smart boy. The first two letters of the alphabet and 1, 2 were about all he could remember after his illness. His behavior at mealtime was not the same either. He would throw food, scream and tear his napkin to pieces. His parents made an appointment and brought him to the clinic. Through NTT we found that he was allergic to the DPT vaccine. We treated him through his mother. After the basic ten, he was treated for DPT. His mother called the clinic the next day to say he was acting even worse than usual, screaming and yelling. He had failed the treatment for the diphtheria component of DPT. We treated him again three more times on three consecutive days for diphtheria. His symptoms subsided immediately. Twenty-five hours after the last treatment, his mother knew he had passed: Ricky was counting to ten again. His hyperactivity subsided, his attention span increased, and he loved to hear his mother read his favorite story.

Pertussis

Pertussis (Whooping Cough) is an acute highly communicable bacterial disease characterized by a cough that usually ends in a prolonged, high-pitched, crowing sound (the whoop). It is transmitted through the air and is found throughout the world. It has increased in the US since the late 1980's. Symptoms begin with sneezing, anorexia, listlessness and a hacking nocturnal cough. The number of coughs increase (5-15 coughs at a time) with mucous, vomiting, and gagging. Approximately one-third of the cases reported to the Center for Disease Control are in infants less than six months old. In infants choking spells may be more common than whoops. Respiratory complications are common, including asphyxia in infants. Residual emphysema, edema, mental retardation, convulsions, and cerebral hemorrhage may result. DPT immunizations are routinely given in the US.

It is important to test the infant for allergy to the DPT immunization before administering it. If the infant is allergic he/she should be treated before the immunization.

NAET HELP

Children can be tested by NTT to see if they would react to the vaccine before being inoculated. If the child is found to be allergic to the vaccine, he/she should be treated using NAET before being inoculated.

If the child is manifesting acute symptoms within hours of injection, provide acute NAET care using a fresh sample of vaccine, or any of the body secretions if the vaccine is not available: saliva, urine, vomit or blood.

If the child is having after effects of vaccination, follow the classic NAET protocol with a practitioner.

Then collect samples of the daily foods in a test tube and treat the child with NAET.

Treat DPT vaccine and all combinations with NAET

ACUHELP: LI-11, SP-10, PC-6 and Kid-6.

Supplements

Calcium lactate 1 pill four times a day.

B vitamins 100 mgs daily in devided doses.

Betaine HCL 1 pill, twice daily.

Multizyme 1 capsule twice a day after meals.

Allerplex 1 cap once or twice daily as needed.

Antioxidant 1 daily.

Essential fatty acid 1 daily.

Measles

A highly contagious, acute viral infection characterized by fever, cough, conjunctivitis, spots, and a spreading rash. Measles is extremely communicable and is spread mainly by small droplets from the nose, throat, and mouth of a person in the early stages of the disease. After a 7-14 day incubation period, measles usually begins with a fever, hacking cough, and conjunctivitis. Spots appear 2 days later; then a rash. At the peak of the illness the fever may be as high as 104 degrees. Measles vaccinations are given in the US. Severe allergic reactions have been reported from this vaccination. Various nervous disorders have surfaced from vaccination allergy including Autism, ADD, ADHD, and learning disabilities. Please read the books, "Say Good-bye To Allergy-related Autism" and "Say Good-bye to ADD and ADHD" by the author if anyone is interested to learn more about ADD, ADHD and Autism.

NAET HELP

Children can be tested by NTT to see if they would react to the vaccine before being inoculated. If the child is found to be allergic to the vaccine, he/she should be treated using NAET before being inoculated.

If the child is manifesting acute symptoms within hours of injection, provide acute NAET care using a fresh sample of vaccine, or any of the body secretions if the vaccine is not available: saliva, urine, vomit or blood.

If the child is having after effects of vaccination, follow the classic NAET protocol with a practitioner.

Then collect samples of the daily foods in a test tube and treat the child with NAET.

Treat MMR vaccine and all combinations with NAET
ACUHELP: LI-11, SP-10, PC-6 and Kid-6.

Supplements

Calcium lactate 1 pill four times a day to reduce fever.

B vitamins 100 mgs daily in devided doses.

Betaine HCL 1 pill, twice daily.

Multizyme 1 capsule twice a day after meals.

Allerplex 1 cap once or twice daily as needed.

Antioxidant 1 daily.

Essential fatty acid 1 daily.

Milk of magnesia or calamine lotion locally.

Vinegar bath to reduce itching in active cases.

Hibiscus tea 1 cup twice a day to eliminate toxins and promote healing.

Mumps

An acute contagious, generalized viral disease, usually causing painful enlargement of the salivary glands. Mumps is endemic in certain heavily populated areas but may occur in epidemics when many susceptible people are crowded together. It is less communicable than measles and chickenpox. The disease may occur at any age, but most cases occur in children aged 5-10 years. The onset of mumps occurs with chills, headache, anorexia, malaise, and a low to moderate fever that may last 12-24 hours before the salivary glands begin to swell. Pain when chewing and swallowing with temperature as high as 103-104 degrees are common. A soft diet reduces the pain caused by chewing. Citrus fruit and acidic substances should be avoided. The American Academy of Pediatrics recommends vaccination with measles-mumps-rubella at 12-15 months of age and again when entering grade school and high school.

NAET HELP

Children can be tested by NTT to see if they would react to the vaccine before being inoculated. If the child is found to be allergic to the vaccine, he/she should be treated using NAET before being inoculated.

If the child is manifesting acute symptoms within hours of injection, provide acute NAET care using a fresh sample of vaccine, or any of the body secretions if the vaccine is not available: saliva, urine, vomit or blood.

If the child is having after effects of vaccination, follow the classic NAET protocol with a practitioner.

Then collect samples of the daily foods in a test tube and treat the child with NAET.

Treat MMR vaccine and all combinations with NAET
ACUHELP: LI-11, SP-10, PC-6 and Kid-6.

Supplements

Calcium lactate 1 pill (Std.process lab.) four times a day.
B vitamins 100 mgs daily in devided doses.
Betaine HCL 1 pill, twice daily.
Multizyme 1 capsule twice a day after meals.
Allerplex 1 cap once or twice daily as needed.
Antioxidant 1 daily.
Essential fatty acid 1 daily.
Epsom salt fomentation to reduce swelling of the glands.

Rubella

(German Measles; three-day Measles)

A contagious viral infection that may result in abortion, stillbirth, or congenital defects in infants born to mothers infected during the early months of pregnancy. After natural infection, immunity appears to last a lifetime. Tender, swollen glands, a rash similar to measles, a low-grade infection, and a red pharynx are symptoms of rubella.

NAET HELP

Children can be tested by NTT to see if they would react to the vaccine before being inoculated. If the child is found to be allergic to the vaccine, he/she should be treated using NAET before being inoculated.

If the child is manifesting acute symptoms within hours of injection, provide acute NAET care using a fresh sample of vaccine, or any of the body secretions if the vaccine is not available: saliva, urine, vomit or blood.

If the child is having after effects of vaccination, follow the classic NAET protocol with a practitioner.

Treat DPT vaccine and all combinations with NAET
ACUHELP: LI-11, SP-10, PC-6 and Kid-6.

Supplements

Calcium lactate 1 pill (standard process lab of so. Ca.) four times a day.

B vitamins 100 mgs daily in devided doses.

Betaine HCL 1 pill, twice daily.

Multizyme 1 capsule twice a day after meals.

Allerplex 1 cap once or twice daily as needed.

Antioxidant 1 daily.

Essential fatty acid 1 daily.

Chickenpox

Chickenpox is extremely contagious and is spread directly by air or contact with the blisters, or indirectly through freshly soiled articles during the early stages of the eruption. When the final lesions have crusted, the patient can no longer transmit the disease. Isolation for six days after the first vesicles appear is usually sufficient to control cross infection. 11-15 days after exposure, mild headache, moderate fever, and general malaise, accompanied by a characteristic rash (crop of blisters). The rash usually begins on the trunk and then spreads to the face and scalp. Most reported cases occur between the ages of 5 and 9. The disease is usually more severe in infants (less than 3 months old), adolescents, and adults. Outbreaks of chickenpox tend to occur from January to June.

NAET HELP

Children can be tested by NTT to see if they would react to the vaccine before being inoculated. If the child is found to be allergic to the vaccine, he/she should be treated using NAET before being inoculated.

If the child is manifesting acute symptoms within hours of injection, provide acute NAET care using a fresh sample of vaccine, or any of the body secretions if the vaccine is not available: saliva, urine, vomit or blood.

If the child is having after effects of vaccination, or regular outbreak of chickenpox, follow the classic NAET protocol with a practitioner.

Treat Chickenpox vaccine or a sample of pox secretion collected from the child's pox in a test tube (Use a Q-tip to collect the sample).

ACUHELP: LI-11, SP-10, PC-6.

Supplements

Calcium lactate 1 pill four times a day.
B vitamins 100 mgs daily in devided doses.
Vitamin C supplements.
Allerplex 1 cap once or twice daily as needed.
Essential fatty acid 1 pill daily.
Milk of magnesia or calamine lotion locally.
Vinegar bath to reduce itching in active cases.

Urinary Tract Infection

A normal urinary tract is usually sterile, even though it may become contaminated with bacteria. In an abnormal urinary tract many organisms can cause infection. E. Coli causes more than 75% of urinary tract infections in all pediatric age groups. In newborns, 1-2 percent develop urinary tract infections, with boys 5 times more likely to have UTI than girls. 5% of school-age children get UTI. The symptoms include diarrhea, vomiting, mild jaundice, lethargy, fever, hypothermia, abdominal pain, cystitis, chills, urinary retention, urgency, pain, and tenderness. UTI can be a symptom of an allergic reaction and treating for a specific bacteria using NTT can be helpful. Laboratory can help you isolate the specific bacteria from urine sample.

NAET HELP

Using NTT, find the causative agent and treat with NAET.

If the child is manifesting acute symptoms and unable to track down the causative agent, provide acute NAET care using a fresh sample of any of the body secretions: saliva, urine, vomit or blood.

If the child is suffering from chronic infection or inflammation, treat him/her using classic NAET protocol.

Collect samples of the daily foods in a test tube and treat the child with NAET.

Treat a sample of urine four times daily in the house.

ACUHELP: LI-11, SP-10, Kid-3, Kid-7, PC-6.

Supplements

Minor cinnamon and peony formula 1 twice a day.

Adequate amount of water to drink.

Agastache formula 1 pill twice daily with meals.

Calcium lactate 1 pill four times a day to reduce fever.

Cranberry juice or pill twice a day after checking for allergy.

Betaine HCL 1 pill, twice daily.

Multizyme 1 capsule twice a day after meals.

Allerplex 1 cap once or twice daily as needed.

Vinegar sitz bath once a day.

Check for an allergy to food, drinks, dtergent, soap, new fabrics, any new medication, vitamins, and supplements.

Hearing Deficits in Children

Hearing loss can happen at any time. 1/800-1/1000 newborns have severe to profound hearing loss at birth. Two to three times as many are born with lesser hearing losses. During childhood, another 2-3/1000 children acquire moderate to severe progressive or permanent hearing loss. Many adolescents are at risk for sensorineural hearing loss from excessive exposure to noise and from head trauma. Hearing deficits in childhood can result in lifelong impairments in receptive and expressive skills.

The most common hearing deficits are acquired conductive losses. Almost every child experiences mild to moderate, intermittent or continual hearing loss from otitis media. Repeated or severe infections can lead to hearing loss. Children most affected by otitis media are those with immune deficiencies, cleft palate, and exposure to environmental risk factors (tobacco smoke, day care placement). Boys are more often affected than girls. Autoimmune disorders, bacterial meningitis, viral infections, rubella, mumps, and sound trauma (loud music, firearms) may cause sensorineural hearing loss.

NAET HELP

Find the causative agent and treat or avoid the allergen.

Treat for classic NAET groups.

Collect samples of daily food and treat at bedtime.

Check grown-up children for the ear phones, ear plugs, new computer, celluar phone, fabrics, new toys, walkie-talkie, new pets, animals, birds, etc.

ACUHELP: TW-5

Earache and Ear Infection

Earaches and infections are common in young children, especially those between the ages of 3 months and three years.

Middle Ear Infection

Middle ear infection is common among little children. The middle ear space where nerves and small bones connect to the eardrum on one side and the eustachian tube on the other side is involved. Middle-ear infection affects all ages but is most common in infants and children.

Signs and symptoms of middle-ear infections include: irritability, earache, feeling of fullness in the child's ear, hearing loss, fever, discharge or leakage from the ear, diarrhea, and children often pulling at the ear.

Possible Causes

• Bacterial or viral infections which spread to the middle ear by way of the eustachian tube may be one of the causes. Child may have had an upper respiratory infection just before getting the middle-ear infection.

• Food allergy may be another cause.

• Sinus and eustachian tube blockage caused by nasal allergies or enlarged adenoids in your child should be checked into.

• A ruptured eardrum may be another possibility.

NAET HELP

Using NTT, find the causative agent and treat with NAET.

If the child is manifesting acute symptoms and unable to track down the causative agent, provide acute NAET care using a fresh sample of any of the body secretions: wax or discharge from the ear if any, saliva, urine, vomit or blood.

If the child is suffering from chronic infection or inflammation, treat him/her using classic NAET protocol.

Collect samples of the daily foods in a test tube and treat the child with NAET.

ACUHELP: LI-11, Liv-3, Kid-3, Kid-7, PC-6.

Supplements

Adequate amount of water to drink.

Agastache formula 1 pill twice daily with meals.
Calcium lactate 1 pill four times a day.
Betaine HCL 1 pill, twice daily.
Multizyme 1 capsule twice a day after meals.
Allerplex 1 cap once or twice daily as needed.

Outer Ear Infection

Outer ear infection is the infection or inflammation of the ear canal that extends from the eardrum to the outside. The skin of the ear canal is involved.

Signs and Symptoms

Ear pain that worsens when the child's earlobe is pulled. Child may have slight fever, discharge or pus from the ear and sometimes temporary loss of hearing on the affected side.

Possible Causes

• Allergy to certain food, drinks, swimming pool water, chlorinated water, ear cleaning objects like Q-tips, etc.
• Bacteria or fungal infection of the delicate skin lining of the child's ear canal. Any of these below may trigger an infection.
• Swimming in dirty, polluted water.
• Excessive swimming in chlorinated water.
• Chlorinated water dries out the ear canal, allowing bacteria or mold to enter the skin.
• Irritation from Q-tips, swabs, cleaning chemicals, playing with foreign objects like bobby pin, pencil, pen, or using ear plugs for longer period.

NAET HELP

Using NTT, find the causative agent and treat with NAET.
If the child is manifesting acute symptoms and unable to track down the causative agent, provide acute NAET care using a fresh

sample of any of the body secretions: wax or discharge from the ear if any, saliva, urine, vomit or blood.

If the child is suffering from chronic infection or inflammation, treat him/her using classic NAET protocol.

Collect samples of the daily foods in a test tube and treat the child with NAET.

ACUHELP: LI-11, Liv-3, Kid-3, Kid-7, PC-6.

Supplements

Adequate amount of water to drink.

Agastache formula 1 pill twice daily with meals.

Calcium lactate 1 pill four times a day.

Betaine HCL 1 pill, twice daily.

Multizyme 1 capsule twice a day after meals.

Allerplex 1 cap once or twice daily as needed.

Conjunctivitis

Conjunctivitis occurs usually due to some kind of allergies. It is an inflammation of the conjunctiva, the delicate membrane that covers the inner eyelid and the external surface of the eye. In most people allergic conductivities is part of a large allergy syndrome, such as seasonal allergic rhinitis. Allergic conjunctivitis can also occur alone in some people who have direct contact with airborne substances like pollens, dusts, fungal spores, animal dander. The white of the eye may turn red, itch and may water a great deal. The eyelid may become swollen and red also. Sensitization, exposure to an antigen that results in hypersensitivity reaction, allergy to medication, allergy to soap, talcum powder, etc., can also cause inflammation of the eye.

Food allergy affecting lung meridian can result in conjunctivitis since the nerve energy to the white of an eye is supplied by lung meridian. Other causes of conjunctivitis are chemical injury, bacterial infection, and viral infection.

NAET HELP

Using NTT, find the causative agent and treat with NAET. If the child is suffering from chronic infection or inflammation, treat him/her using classic NAET protocol.

Collect samples of the daily foods in a test tube and treat the child with NAET.

ACUHELP: LI-11, Liv-3, Kid-3, Kid-7, PC-6.

Supplements

Adequate amount of water to drink.
Agastache formula 1 pill twice daily with meals.
Calcium lactate 1 pill four times a day.
Iplex 1 tablet two times a day
Occulotrophin 1 tablet two times a day
Allerplex 1 cap once or twice daily as needed.
Breast milk is a popular old-time remedy for conjunctivitis. A drop of breast milk instilled every 3-4 hours for a couple of days can give some relief to the sufferer.

But if the causative agent can be detected through NTT, and the allergy eliminated through NAET, child's conjuntivitis can be brought under control in just a few minutes to hours.

Pinworm Infestation

Pinworms are parasites that invade the gastrointestinal tract. They affect approximately 20% of the children 5-10 years old. They cause anal itching that is usually worse at night. Enterobius is the most common parasite infesting children in temperate climates. It is transmitted by hand to mouth and is not related to personal hygiene. Close contact is required for transmission. Toys, clothing, towels, bed sheets, and furniture can transmit the pinworms. The infection is more common in late fall and early winter. The pinworms reach maturity in the lower GI tract within 2-6 weeks. Multiple infestations of members within a household often occur so treatment of all family members is necessary. The usual treatment is mebendazole and a cream or ointment to stop the itching. Re-infestation commonly occurs. Pinworms can be treated by NAET to eliminate them from recurring.

NAET HELP

First treat for NAET group-C. Then treat by priority.

Collect samples of the daily foods in a test tube and treat the child with NAET.

Collect a sample of stool and treat daily.

Treat for NAET group-A, then for parasites and pinworms, then treat by priority.

ACUHELP: LI-11, SP-6, ST-35.

Supplements

Adequate amount of water to drink.

Calcium lactate 1 pill four times a day.

Betaine HCL 1 pill, twice daily.

Multizyme 1 capsule twice a day between meals.

Pancreatic enzyme 1 daily between meals.

Allerplex 1 cap once or twice daily as needed.

Cystic Fibrosis

Cystic fibrosis is a familial disease primarily affecting the GI and respiratory systems. Chronic obstructive lung disease, pancreatic deficiency, and elevated concentration of salts in the sweat characterize CF. It is the most common severe inherited disease in the white population and occurs in 1 out of every 2500 Caucasians; 1 out of 17,000 African-Americans; and is rarely seen in Asians. 70% of the patients are children. In infants, at onset of the disease, there may be a delay in regaining birth weight and inadequate weight gain from 4-6 weeks of age. 50% of the patients have pulmonary symptoms, usually chronic cough and wheezing with recurrent or chronic pulmonary infections, and a barrel chest. Coughing, gagging, vomiting and disturbed sleep are the most common complaints. Adolescents may have retarded growth, delayed onset of puberty, and a declining tolerance for exercise. Pancreatic functions are severely impaired in 85-90% of the patients. Clinical manifestations may be related to a deficiency of fat-soluble vitamins. The prognosis has improved steadily over the past 50 years, because of aggressive treatment before the onset of irreversible pulmonary changes.

NAET HELP
Treat for classic NAET groups, individual vitamin C groups, individual minerals, individual amino acids, fatty acids, and individual bacteria.
ACUHELP: St-36, SP-6, LI-11, Liv-3, Kid-3, SP-9.

My Child's Cystic Fibrosis

Dear Linda,

I am writing to give you an update on Marcy since we last saw you. As you know, I have been bringing Marcy to see you since the end of July this year to receive NAET treatment for the alleviation of her symptoms due to cystic fibrosis. Marcy has had sparse pseudomonas bacterial growth in her lungs since August of 1998 (last year). She has had mild cough and phlegm in the back of her throat as a result of the excess mucus production due to pseudomonas.

We entered a new territory by treating her for pseudomonas with NAET and strengthening her lungs with acupressure based on the NAET system. Well, after only a few sessions with you, I was thrilled when Marcy's throat culture, taken at the end of

August, came back negative, indicating that the pseudomonas was gone. Shortly after the culture results, Marcy's cough was gone as well. The last three weeks have been very exciting and promising for us. Marcy's doctor, a pediatric pulmonologist specializing in Cystic Fibrosis, said Marcy had a 50/50 chance of completely getting rid of the pseudomonas; we always knew it was possible and now we are so happy to experience this tremendous sense of relief.

Thank you Linda, for your willingness to work with children, to learn and try new ways of treatment and for being a part of Marcy's healing process. Marcy and I are looking forward to seeing you soon and continuing our wonderful treatment. I know she has a long way to go before she can conquer all her allergies. But now I have hope that she is going to be a normal child when she completes her treatment program.

Yours Truly,

Sue Ann (signed)

NAET Practitioner: *Linda Miyoshi, L.Ac*
Bethesda, Maryland 20814

Hypoglycemia

Hypoglycemia, (blood glucose<40mg/dL) usually occurs because the child is born with a defective glycogen storage mechanism. Listlessness, poor feeding, apnea, or seizures may occur. Neonatal hypoglycemia can lead to neurological damage so it should be treated promptly.

NAET HELP

Treat for NAET group-A, acid, base, insulin, pancreas, liver, inositol, and sugar with all basic combinations.

Collect a sample of the baby formula (any other food the child is eating) in a test tube and treat the child.

Collect samples of foods taken during the day and treat using self-help points before bedtime.
ACUHELP: SP-6, ST-36.

Supplements
Betaine hydrochloric acid 1 twice a day.
Multizyme 1 once a day.
Paraplex 1 twice a day
Pancreatin 1 twice daily
Drenamin 1 once a day
Adequate amount of water to drink.

Withdrawal from Drugs
(Cocaine, opioids, and barbiturates)

Infants born to addicted mothers have low birth weight, reduced body length and head circumference. Some newborns show withdrawal symptoms if the mother used drugs before delivery. Characteristic signs include irritability, internal tremors, vomiting, diarrhea, sweating, convulsions, mental fog, and hyperventilation. The incidence of SIDS is greater in infants born to narcotic addicts.

NAET HELP
Treat NAET group- A and supplement with B vitamins, vitamin A, and organic minerals.

Treat for the samples of the drugs taken by the mother.

Then treat for the rest of the classic NAET groups by priority.
ACUHELP: LIV-5, LI-4.

Seizure Disorders

Seizures are a frequent and sometimes serious neonatal problem. Infections, pesticides, parasites, formaldehyde, latex allergy, food colors and food additives can cause seizures. Seizures are frequent with meningitis, herpes simplex virus, and rubella virus.

NAET HELP

Treat NAET group-A and supplement with B vitamins and trace minerals.

Treat for everyday food groups.

Treat for pesticides, parasites, formaldehyde, latex allergy, food colors and food additives, then treat the rest of the classic group by priority.

Sudden Infant Death Syndrome

The sudden and unexpected death of any infant or child in which a thorough postmortem examination fails to show an adequate cause. SIDS causes 30% of all deaths between the ages of 2 weeks and one year. Most deaths occur between the second and fourth months of life. Lower socioeconomic groups, premature infants, and infants born to mothers who smoke during pregnancy are at greater risk of SIDS. Almost all SIDS deaths occur when the infant is thought to be sleeping.

Although the cause of SIDS is unknown, it is most likely due to dysfunction of neural cardiorespiratory control mechanisms. Many studies suggest that a prone sleeping position, soft bedding (lamb's wool), water bed mattresses, smoking in the home, and an overheated environment may increase the risk of SIDS.

The American Academy of Pediatrics recommends that infants be placed supine for sleep unless other medical conditions prevent this. Every effort should be made to avoid an overheated environment; to avoid over-wrapping the infant; to remove soft bedding, pillows, or comforters from the crib; and to avoid smoking during and after pregnancy.

In our experience, children are allergic to the materials used on the crib. Chemicals, formaldehyde, fabrics and latex are some of the culprits.

NAET HELP

Find the causative agent(s) and treat.

Avoid using anything on the infant before checking for possible allergies; if found eliminate them before use.

Sudden Infant Death Syndrome

Eddie was one week old when his mother found him in his crib without any signs of life. She shook him. He wasn't breathing. Her husband called the paramedics. Three minutes later the paramedics arrived. Eddie's heart had stopped. They used a defibrillator to revive him. He was taken to the hospital and was monitored for 48 hours. The hospital sent a beeping monitor home with his parents. If Eddie stopped breathing the monitor would go off. The beeper went off several times a day. He would be fine in the hospital, but had difficulty breathing at home. After testing all the items in his crib we found that Eddie was allergic to the plastic bumper guard and plastic accessories around his crib. His breathing difficulties stopped after he was treated for those items by NAET.

Juvenile Rheumatoid Arthritis

Arthritis beginning at or before the age of sixteen is referred to as juvenile rheumatoid arthritis. It affects the large and small joints and may interfere with growth and development. Therapy is similar to adults but aspirin is not recommended in the USA because of concern about Reye's syndrome, Ibuprofen or Naproxen is given instead. Complete remissions occur in 50-75% of the patients. Juvenile Rheumatoid Arthritis affects approximately 70,000 children in the USA and affects girls twice as often as it affects boys. Symptoms include pain, inflammation, and stiffness in one or more joints, which may appear suddenly. Morning and late afternoon or evening stiffness that improves after a hot shower/bath or with stretching and mild exercise is another common symptom of JRA. Patients with JRA may also have eye pain, redness, enlarged spleen, and a salmon colored skin rash.

NAET HELP

Treat for NAET classic groups.

Treat for daily-food-samples.

Treat for body secretions, urine, blood, individual bacteria, organs, specific tissues of involvement at the site of discomfort. (muscles, nerve tissue, elastin, collagen, osteocast, osteoblast, immunoglobulins (IgA, IgE, IgG, IgM) glands, hormones, find individual bacteria (either by QRT or run a carbon based test or ALCAT test for bacteria), parasite, fungus, virus, vaccines, pesticides, formaldehyde, synthetic materials, detergent, other chemicals, any drugs taken in the past or present, emotional blockages, arthritic factor, and any combinations found.

Supplements

Siler and platycodon 1 twice a day.

Drenamine 1 pill three times a day.

Betaine hydrochloric acid 1 pill twice a day.

Multizyme 1capsule twice a day.

Allergy to Millet

Sandy could not get dressed for school without her mother's help each morning because her joint pain was so severe. It was difficult for her to hold a pencil and write at school. With exercise the swelling would subside for a while but would return before dinner. By the time her mother brought her to see us, Sandy was missing one or two days of school a week because she couldn't get out of bed in the morning. We found that she was highly allergic to the millet cereal she was eating for breakfast every morning that her mother bought at the health food store. After she was treated for grains and millet with NAET her joint pains disappeared.

Camy had a different problem. She was diagnosed as arthritic 9 months ago. She was on disability. When we saw her in our office, through NTT, it was revealed that she was allergic to her birth control pills which was the cause of her pain. She had begun taking the pill 9 moths ago. Immediately she was treated for the pill. Her pain continued for 45 hours, during that time she massaged her general balancing points hourly. At the end of 45 hours after the treatment, her pain relieved completely.

Erica woke up crying with swollen, painful hands. She never had symptoms like that before. Her mother was a patient of ours and brought her to our clinic immediately. The five-year-old's fingers were twice their normal size. She couldn't move them or hold anything in her hands. She was also having pains in her feet and her body ached all over. We traced the problem to corn she had eaten the day before. She ate corn flakes at breakfast, some corn bread with lunch, and had corn on the cob with her dinner. We treated her for corn and the swelling in her hands began to subside almost immediately. After the twenty-five hour period her joint pain and swelling were completely gone and hasn't returned in five years.

Autism

This is an early childhood syndrome characterized by abnormal social relationships; language disorder with impaired understanding, pronominal reversal; rituals and compulsive phenomena; and uneven intellectual development. Autism is two to four times more common in boys than girls, and usually manifests itself in the first-third year of life. Extreme aloofness (failure to cuddle, avoidance of eye gaze); insistence on sameness (rituals, repeated acts, and resistance to change); speech and language disorders (total muteness to idiosyncratic use of language), and uneven intellectual performance characterize the syndrome. Symptoms tend to remain constant throughout development with some individuals acquiring symptoms of schizophrenia in adolescence or young adulthood. Behavior therapy helps manage the child in the home and at school. Several psychotropic drugs have been used, but there is little evidence of their effectiveness. Speech therapy should begin early. Children with near normal or higher IQ's often benefit from special education. Autistic children treated with NAET have made excellent progress in their behavior, speech, learning, and socialization skills. Autistic children have difficulty breaking down milk protein and undigested protein might get into the circulation and to the brain causing irritability and abnormal behaviors. After successful NAET treatments, the body will learn to make the appropriate digestive enzymes to break down the proteins. Please also read "Say Good-bye to Allergy-related Autism" by the author. This book has much valuable information to take care of your autistic child.

Schizophrenia

Childhood schizophrenia forms a continuum with adolescent and adult forms. It is characterized by withdrawal, apathy, thought disorder (blocking and perseverance), hallucinations and delusions.

Specialized educational systems may be required because this disorder significantly affects the child's development. Combined psychotropic and psychotherapeutic treatment may be required. Residential treatment has become rare in the USA so that family members, friends, and social agencies have to provide care.

NAET HELP

Using NTT find the causative agent if possible and avoid the substance or get treated by NAET for the allergen.

Treat for classic NAET groups.

Treat individual amino acids and neurotransmitters.

Treat the samples of daily diet.

Continue all other treatments.

B vitamins, especially B-6, trace minerals, supplements

Simplex M for boys and simplex F for girls (from Stad. process lab) 1 tablet twice a day.

Minchex 1 cap twice a day.

ACUHELP: St-36, SP-6, Liv-5, GV 20, HT-7 and Kid-6.

Childhood Depression

The basic manifestations of childhood depression are similar to those seen in adults but are related to typical concerns of children, such as schoolwork and play. A sad appearance, apathy, withdrawal, feeling rejected and unloved, headaches, abdominal pains, clowning or foolish behavior, and persistent self-blame. Chronic depressive reactions are associated with anorexia, weight loss, despondency, and suicidal thoughts. Extremes of irritability and aggression, rather than a depressed mood are quite common. In some cases childhood depression may turn into bipolar disorder later on in life. The family and social setting needs to be evaluated to determine the stresses that may have triggered the depression. The family and school need to focus on enhancing the child's self-esteem.

NAET HELP

Treat for classic NAET groups.
Treat individual amino acids.
Supplement adequate amino acids.
In addition, D-phenylalanine 1 twice daily.
Inositol 1 twice a day.
Choline 1 tab twice a day.
Drenamin 1 pill three times a day.

Depression

Erin, ten-years-old, was having difficulty sleeping through the night. She would get up two to three times and couldn't fall back to sleep. She became depressed and stopped participating in school. She didn't want to socialize or play with her friends. The school counselor, her teacher, and her mother could not get her to snap out of her depression and sleeplessness. She was allergic to many foods, but it wasn't until we tested and treated her for serotonin (a neurotransmitter) that she was able to sleep through the night.

Mild Depression

This occurs in at least 10% of high school students, moderate depression in 5-6% and major depression in 1-2%. Genetics plays a significant part in adolescent depression. If the parents suffered from depression, most likely the children could get it too, probably would start at an earlier date. The cause of more than half of adolescent suicidal behaviors is depression. The symptoms are similar to adult depression, but may be modified by circumstances in the adolescent's life. Younger adolescents may not be able to explain inner feelings or moods or older adolescents may feel it is weak to do so. Depression should be considered when a previously well performing student withdraws from society or commits delinquent acts.

A twelve-year-old boy was diagnosed as being clinically depressed. He had failing grades at school, was irritable, disruptive and belligerent in school and at home. The doctor prescribed antidepressants, but nothing seemed to help. He was referred to our office and found to be allergic to pesticides, detergents, soaps, sugars, and grains. After he was cleared of allergies he was given large doses of B complex vitamins. When his B complex requirement was met, he no longer needed any antidepressants and his behavior became normal.

Post-traumatic Stress Disorder

Posttraumatic Stress Disorder may follow major traumatic events (natural or man-made disasters) immediately or after several weeks' delay, even in generally stable youth. Adults commonly underestimate the effects of these events on children and may not spend enough time discussing them. Reassuring the child is very important and the parents and guardians should be comforting and supportive. Individual, family and group therapy is helpful.

NAET HELP

Treat for classic NAET groups.
Treat the samples of everyday meals.
B vitamins, especially B-12 1000mcg three times a day.

Substance Abuse Disorders

Substance abuse is the repeated use of drugs with adverse consequences. It has penetrated all age groups, including preadolescents. Daily use of marijuana and experimentation with a variety of compounds varies from year to year, but alcohol remains the principal substance of abuse. Heroin, cocaine, crack cocaine, and other stimulant abuse is less common but also significant in children and adolescents. No matter the type of drug the symptoms remain the same in substance abuse. The child or adolescent is less engaged in school, more interested in recreation, and more likely to have a job and money. There is a progression from alcohol and tobacco to marijuana and then other compounds. Alcohol abuse rises in mid-to-late adolescents. Most people begin serious abuse before the age of twenty. Tobacco use usually predicts the abuse of other substances.

NAET has been successful in treating alcohol, tobacco, and substance abuse disorders because they involve allergy.

NAET HELP

Treat for classic NAET groups.
Treat the substances used by the mother.

Bipolar Disorder
(Manic-depressive psychosis)

It is rare for children to have severe mood swings before puberty, but it does occur. Depression in adolescents often signals the beginning of bipolar disorder. Mania in adolescents is commonly confused with schizophrenia. It is the cyclical pattern of depression and mania that indicates bipolar disorder. Bipolar disorders have been traced back to some allergies and NAET treatment has been successful in many cases.

NAET HELP

Treat for classic NAET groups.
Check for the family members' allergy; if found treat them.
Treat all samples of food products.

Behavioral Problems

Knowing when a behavior is difficult but normal or a problem is not always easy. A significant problem is more likely when the behavior is frequent and chronic, when more than one problem behavior occurs, and particularly when the behavior interferes with social and cognitive functioning. Many problem behaviors are typical of certain stages of development (oppositional behavior in a two-year-old). The health developmental stage and temperament of the child should be assessed. A log of the child's activities each day should be kept. Direct observations of the parent and child interaction often provide clues to the behavior. Observations by teachers, relatives and friends give additional insight into the problem. An allergy may be the cause of the problem. Testing and treating with NAET will eliminate the food allergies and the behavioral problems.

NAET HELP

Treat for classic NAET groups.
Check for the family members' allergy if found treat them.
Treat all samples of food products.

Eating Disorders

Parents of young children often complain that they are not eating enough food or eating the wrong foods. Forcing a child to eat usually is detrimental. The child may sit with food in his/her mouth or vomit it up. Continued coercion or over concern may lead to eating problems and disorders. Parents should not become emotional at mealtime. Food should be removed after twenty minutes or so without discussing what was not eaten. Mealtimes should be pleasant, happy occasions. An allergy may be the cause of the problem. Testing and treating with NAET will eliminate the food allergies.

Sleep Disorders

Three to four-year-olds, in particular, have trouble differentiating fantasy from reality. Nightmares can be caused by frightening experiences (scary stories, television violence). An occasional nightmare is normal; however, frequent or persistent nightmares should be discussed with your physician. Night terrors (sudden awakening with screaming and panic) usually occur in the first few hours of sleep, in children from three to eight-years-old. If the episodes continue into adolescence an underlying psychological disorder should be considered. Awakening during the night occurs in about 50% of infants 6-12 months old. In older children episodes often follow a stressful event (illness, divorce). Allowing the child to sleep with the parents usually prolongs the problem. Returning the child to bed and comforting him/her is usually more effective. An allergy may be the cause of the problem. Testing and treating with NAET will eliminate the food allergies.

Bedwetting

Adam, five-years-old, was always running to the bathroom. His kindergarten teacher called his mother to complain that he was having too many accidents in class. At night he would wet his bed. His mother thought that he would grow out of it. We tested him and found he was allergic to the iodized salt. His mother told us that Adam loved salty foods and always wanted to eat pretzels and potato chips. They were his favorite snacks. After he cleared for iodized salt Adam's bed-wetting and urinary problems disappeared.

Hyperactivity

Hyperactivity is not easily defined because it reflects the tolerance level of the annoyed person. More active children with short attention spans create problems for their peers and for adults. Two-year-old children are usually active and four-year-olds have a high activity and noise level. However, extreme hyperactive behavior may be a sign of an emotional disorder, an allergic reaction, or a genetic component. Please read the book "Say goodbye to ADD and ADHD by the author.

ADD / ADHD An Affective Disorder

Sam R. was a 13-year-old who was doing very poorly in school in spite of the massive doses of Ritalin he received and his parents tutoring him four hours every day. Due to the medication he walked like a zombie with no expression on his face or personality. He was underweight for his age. We found him to be severely allergic to milk and cheese, and was consuming dairy products virtually at every meal. After NAET treatments he was able to get off Ritalin, gained 40 pounds and grew 6 inches in height within the next six months. The following year he won an award for the top math student in his grade in the entire school district, and is making straight A's. As the result of Ralph's "Miracle," over 60 patients have come from his geographical area to be treated at our clinic, an eight hour round trip drive! Without NAET we never would have been able to resurrect Ralph nor the many other patients we have helped with behavior problems, attention deficit disorders, hyperactivity, and emotional problems. Thank you Dr. Devi from all of us.

Dr. James H. Winer, D.C.
1320 E. Carson St.
Pittsburgh, PA 15203   (412) 431-7246

Sugar Allergy!

Dear Doctor,

I'm writing to let you know how pleased I am by the results of your examination and NAET treatment on my son, Nick, on August 10 through 14, 1998. My son had been diagnosed with attention-deficit hyperactive disorder and was taking Ritalin by prescription from his pediatrician. The Ritalin was not producing the results that I had desired, so, in a desperate attempt to help him, I sought out and turned to a natural method. I had also observed that he did not react well to processed sugar. Specifically, I observed that within 20-30 minutes of drinking soda or eating candy, he became excessively energetic and was unable to focus on anything for more than a few minutes. As you recall, I brought him to you for examination and testing with regards to these problems.

On August 12th, you tested him for allergies to sugar and discovered a strong allergy to sugar... up to a distance of more than five feet! I was present during the testing and personally witnessed the results. If I understood correctly, your test also indicated that his brain was producing too much energy. You performed the NAET procedure which, I'm told, is designed to clear allergies from the body. I was present before and after the procedure. I was not allowed to stand in the same room while he was being treated to avoid the interference with his magnetic field. After his treatment we waited in his office for the next 20 minutes, then my son was asked to wash his hands with plain water to remove the energy of the sugar from his hands.

My son had to abstain from sugar in any form for 25 hours after the procedure was finished in order for it to work. All foods containing sugar, including packaged food, fruit, etc., were put away in closed cabinets, and I followed a list of permitted foods for his diet for the next 25 hours. He was allowed to eat white rice, vegetables, chicken, eggs, vegetable oil, and salt. And he was allowed to drink water. Honestly, Doctor, it wasn't easy, but we survived the 25 hours. And now? Well, without any hesitation, I am ecstatic with the results! The day after the procedure was finished for the sugar, my son ate three sweet rolls at church- the kind with the white sugary icing on top. I was completely amazed: he remained completely calm. If this had been two weeks earlier, that much sugar would have left him bouncing like a rubber ball! One of our church members even commented on how "Subdued" Nick had been during the service. She asked if he was tired. I explained to her what we had done at your office. She was a bit surprised, After all, this was the first time she had heard about the NAET procedure. Nevertheless, she said, "Well, it works! So who am I to doubt it?". Doctor, I can't thank you enough. Since that day in Church, I have seen many more instances to corroborate the results of NAET. The bottom line: Nick is no longer allergic to sugar! thank you for the tiny miracle that has made a huge impact on my boy's life.

Thankfully yours,
Happy Mom

An eight-year-old boy was having difficulty in the third grade. He had always had difficulty in school, but his/her teacher felt he was falling too far behind the other students. He wasn't able to follow directions, sit for more than a minute at a time, and would bother the other children while they were working. He wasn't able to read anything but the simplest words. Subtraction was impossible for him to compute. The teacher told his mother that she felt he needed to be tested for a special education class. His hyperactivity was interfering with his schooling. He was a problem at home also, fighting with his little brother, breaking toys or throwing them around the house. Dinner had become a nightmare. Food would be everywhere but on his plate or in his mouth. His mother brought him to the clinic in desperation. She didn't know how to control him anymore, but she didn't want to medicate him as the school had suggested. Testing him we found that he was allergic to sugar. His mother said she rarely gave him sugary products like cookies or candies. But he had to have a certain breakfast cereal every morning and loved fruit. Some nights at dinner he asked to have his cereal. Of course the cereal was loaded with sugar and fruit juice. After clearing for sugars, his behavior improved. His schoolwork was at the third grade level after we completed the treatments for grains, his particular breakfast cereal, and fruits.

Learning Disorders

The inability to acquire, retain, or generalize specific skills or sets of information because of deficiencies in attention, memory, perception, or reasoning is called a learning disorder. A learning disability is a specific learning disorder and refers to a problem in reading, arithmetic, spelling, writing, and in understanding and/ or the use of expressive language and nonverbal abilities.

Mild to moderate learning disorders are usually not recognized until the child enters school. Physical and behavioral signs may appear early in children with learning problems. They often have minor physical abnormalities and communication problems. Many have neurological deficits or delays and problems with large or gross motor coordination. Difficulty learning the names of colors, letters of the alphabet, or counting may be an early sign of a learning disability. Other early signs are short attention span, motor restlessness and distractibility, limited verbal fluency, speech problems, limited memory span, and fine motor problems (poor printing).

Tina was having trouble in preschool. Whenever it was time to color or paint she would become disruptive. She would throw the crayons on the floor or at the other children. She would knock down the easel with all the paints on it. She couldn't identify shapes or colors or count to five or write her name. Her teacher told her mother she was not ready for a school setting. Tina was reacting to the food colorings and food preservatives she was coming in contact with on a daily basis. The coloring in the crayons, chemicals in the paints, the food colorings in the fruit juices and gelatin she had at snack time at preschool caused the learning difficulties. After being treated, she was able to write her name, color, paint, and count to 20 without any difficulty. She also received a good citizen award at the end of the school year.

Attention Deficit Disorder

A persistent and frequent pattern of developmentally inappropriate inattention and impulsivity, with or without hyperactivity. ADD affects 5-10% of school-aged children. ADD tends to occur in families and is common in first-degree relatives. ADD with hyperactivity and impulsivity is seen 10 times more frequently in boys than girls. DSM-IV criteria for ADD include nine signs of inattention, six signs of hyperactivity, and three signs of impulsivity. All signs do not have to be present for a child to have ADD, but the symptoms must be present in two or more situations (at home and at school). The symptoms must impair social and academic functioning. Please read "Say Good-bye to ADD and ADHD" by the author.

HIVES
(Urticaria)

Urticaria or hives is a rash that consists of a single or multiple itchy raised bumps on the skin. It may occur from a reaction to many different stimuli: foods, insect bites, chemicals, clothing, drugs, heat, exercise, or exposure to sunlight. It may subside quickly or be chronic, lasting longer than weeks.

NAET HELP

Treat for the causative agent using NAET.
Treat classic NAET groups.
Allerplex 1 three times a day as needed.
ACUHELP: LI-11, SP-10

Steven's skin would break out in hives and rashes two–three times a week. Cortisone creams and ointments were prescribed, but the hives and rashes kept coming back. He was embarrassed to go to school; the other kids thought his rash was contagious and wouldn't play with him. He had to wear gloves at night to keep from scratching himself until he bled. Checking him through NTT, he was reacting to a food he was eating on a regular basis, at least 2-3 times a week. His mother said that during the last few months she had been trying to have the family eat more fish and vegetables. The only fish Steven would eat was salmon and carrots the only vegetable. Steven tested highly allergic to vitamin A mix and beta-carotene, which includes fish and carrots. His hives and rashes disappeared after he cleared for the NAET group-A food groups, including fish and beta-carotene.

Six-week-old Madison was brought to the office by her mother. Her bottom was raw with an oozing rash. She cried as soon as you touched it. Testing using her mother as a surrogate we found that she was allergic to the plastic diapers that she was wearing. The hives disappeared almost immediately after she cleared for the diapers.

Nancy loved to help her grandma make cookies. She would take all her time to shape the cookies into animals, rolling the dough between her hands. She couldn't wait for Saturday morning to go to her grandma's house to bake. The holidays were the most exciting time. They would make fancy cakes, breads, and pastries. Nancy's hands had been itchy, dry, and scaly for a long time, but right after Christmas they began cracking and developing red bumps all over. Nancy was allergic to yeast, baking powder, flour, and sugar. She was asked to stay away from baking until she was treated for the basic ten food groups, baking powder, and yeast. As she passed her basic ten treatments her hands continue to improve. When she passed the treatment for yeast her hands were no longer itchy, dry, or scaly. The rash has never returned, even during the heavy baking period during the holiday season.

Pre Menstrual Symptom (PMS)

Many youngsters begin their puberty very early, as early as 9 years old. Some children get severe premenstrual disorders. People with PMS also suffer from food craving. Usually they crave sugar, salt, chocolate, spices, hot spices, red meat, etc. They may be allergic to these very things they crave. When they eat these allergic foods they could cause swelling and water retention in the body. Retaining water in the body causes to reduced circulation, and keep the toxins trapped in the body; this will lead to lots of pain and discomfort in the tissue where the toxins are trapped.

NAET HELP

Treating for the NAET group-A usually relieves the problem. Drink lots of water to improve the circulation
Ovotrophin 1 tablet twice a day
Utrophin 1 tablet twice a day

Headaches

There are various types of headaches. They have different causes too. When little children complain of headaches it is usually coming from an allergic reaction to something they ate, drank, touched or inhaled. Allergy to milk, cereals, sugar, books, coloring materials, food additives, clothes, dyes on the clothes, animals and pets, are the major causes. As soon as you find the causes and eliminate them, your child will be free of headaches. If it is due to any other reason (growth, tumor, etc.) you should consult with a neurologist.

Backaches

Very young children usually do not complain of backaches. Their vertebral column is flexible, movable, usually with a lot of disc space. Usually nerve impingement does not happen. When the child grows up into a teenager, the problem begins. If they are allergic to the environmental allergens like grass, pollen, chemicals, paint, perfume, fabrics, sports materials, etc, if the allergens are affecting the kidney meridians, they too can get backaches.

NAET HELP

Find the cause and treat with NAET.
Treat with classic NAET.

Treat for daily-food-samples, and other items from daily use.
ACUHELP: Massage GV-26

Dear Dr Devi,
When I was a little girl I could not wear my shoes and socks;
they would bother me. I used to scream and shout if somebody
told me to wear my shoes. Now that you have treated my allergy
to the shoes I am happy to wear them.
Thank you.

Love,
Devon

Traditional testing procedure are cumbersome and/or painful and may not provide the expected results often. A patch test is complicated since the possibilities of allergens are endless. If at all possible your doctor might do patch tests on one or two allergen at a time; it can take years before one completes the testing alone. NTT offers a better solution in the generalized random screening for the culprit since many items can be tested painlessly and more accurately in a short period of time. NTT can be learned by practitioners and patients alike by understanding the concepts of kinesiology. It is made simple and explained with illustrations in Chapter 7. It is for you to learn it master it to make your life stress-free and disease-free.

The most effective traditional treatment for most allergic conditions and hypersensitivity conditions is avoidance of the substance. Another choice is taking antihistamines and antiinflammatory medications. There is nothing wrong in taking medications where it is necessary. In acute cases one may need to take drugs to control the acute situation faster. Drugs do help to stabilize the condition in a few minutes. But when the acute phase is over, one needs to find ways to prevent future acute attacks. Drugs are chemicals, and can become toxic if you take it too long.

Most of the health problems in children and adults originate from some kind of allergy. If you can find your child's allergy using NTT, you can eliminate them using NAET treatments. NAET may require a number of detailed individual treatments to get the best results. But NAET treatment is known to eliminate the allergies often permanently to the treated item and help your child grow into a healthy, happy adult.

CHAPTER 7

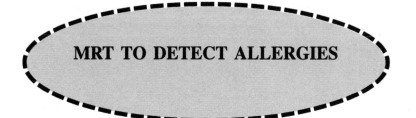

MRT TO DETECT ALLERGIES

7

MUSCLE RESPONSE TESTING

M uscle response testing is one of the tools used by the NAET specialists to test the imbalances and allergies in the body. NAET Muscle Response Testing is developed from applied kinesiology. NAET has much to thank Dr. George Goodheart and associates for developing Muscle Response Testing to detect allergies.

The word "kinesiology" refers to the science of movement. It was first proposed in 1964 by Dr. George Goodheart, a Detroit doctor of chiropractic medicine. As a function of his practice, Dr. Goodheart learned a great deal about a patient's condition by using isolated movements of various muscles. Isolation techniques—a chiropractic procedure, made it possible to test the strength of an individual muscle or muscle group without the help of other muscles. Dr. Goodheart, with the help of Dr. Hetrick and others concluded after many experiments, that structural imbalance causes disorganization of the entire body. This disorganization results in specific disorders of the glands, organs and central nervous system. His findings were similar to what pioneer Chinese doctors also had observed.

Kinesiology holds that when the body is disorganized, the structural balance or electrical force is not functioning normally. When that happens, the electrical energy–life force doesn't flow freely through the nerve cells and causes energy blockages in the person. According to the Chinese, the free flow of energy is necessary for the normal functioning of the body. When your flow of energy gets blocked, you become ill. The messages both from and to the brain also pass through this energy channel. The energy and the messages travel from cell to cell in nanoseconds.

Many years ago, pioneer Chinese doctors and philosophers had studied these energy pathways and networks of the human body energy system by observing living people and their normal and abnormal body functions. The Chinese had learned to manipulate these energy pathways, or meridians, to the body's advantage. About 4,000 years ago, there was no scientific equipment available to feel or observe the presence of the energy flow and its pathways. Now, it is possible to study and trace the energy flows and pathways by using Kirlian photography and radioactive tracer isotopes. Although the existence of energy pathways in the human body has only been confirmed relatively recently, the Chinese doctors hypothesized and established their existence long ago.

Chinese medical theory points out that free-flow of Chi through the meridians is necessary to keep the body in perfect balance. In the United States during the 19th century, the founder of Chiropractic medicine, Daniel David Palmer, said, "Too much or too little energy is sickness." Even though it is believed that Palmer may have had no knowledge of Chinese medicine, his theory corresponded with the ancient Chinese theory of "free flow of energy."

In late 1800's, American chiropractic medicine developed under Dr. D. D. Palmer. Through him, doctors of chiropractic learned about the importance of stabilizing energy and manipulating the spinal segments and nerve roots to keep them perfectly aligned, bringing the body to a balanced state. In the East, acupuncture developed based on the ancient Chinese theory. Eastern acupuncturists tried to bring balance by manipulating the energy meridians at various acupuncture points, inserting needles to remove blockages and reinstating the "free flow of Chi" along the energy pathways. East and West, unaware of each other's findings, worked in a similar manner toward the same goal: to balance the energy and to free sick people from their pain.

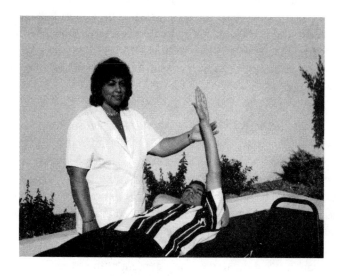

Figure 7-1
Standard Muscle Response Testing

Both groups realized that the overflow or underflow of energy, or in other words, too much or too little energy is the cause of an imbalance. When the flow is reinstated, the balance is restored.

Can You Remove the Blockage?

A trained acupuncturist can differentiate between the overflow and underflow of Chi, and its affected meridians and organs. When treatment is administered to strengthen the under flowing or hypo-functioning organ, while draining the overflowing meridians and the organs, balance is achieved faster. This is the practice of acupuncture. NTT and NAET are built on acupuncture theory, but have taken it one step further. Using the ideas from acupuncture theory, without using actual needle insertion, meridians can be unblocked, overflowing meridians can be drained and the excess energy can be rerouted through the empty meridians and associated organs. Thus the entire body reaches homeostasis. NAET is perhaps the missing link that various professionals have been searching for years. NTT and NAET will be discussed in detail in later chapters.

When the body senses a danger or a threat from an allergen, sensory nerves carry the message to the brain and the brain will alert the whole body about the imminent danger. Muscles contract to conserve energy, other defense forces like lymph, blood cells, etc., get ready to face the emergency. Spinal nerves also get tightened due to the contracted muscles. Vertebrae go into misalignment causing impingement at the affected vertebral level. Energy is blocked due to the impingement. So, a good chiropractic adjustment can remove the nerve impingement at the specific vertebral level and this can unblock the blocked energy pathway making the energy circulate again freely.

Herbs can cause similar healing. Electromagnetic forces of special herbs actually have the ability to enter selective energy pathways and push energy blockages out of the body to restore the energy balance. A well-trained herbologist can bring about the same result as an NAET specialist. Chiropractic, kinesiology, acupuncture and herbology are blended together to create NAET.

NAET treatment works with the entire body: the physical body (organs, brain, nervous system and tissues), physiological body (circulation of blood, fluids and nerve energy) and emotional body (mind, thoughts and spirituality). It helps to detoxify the system

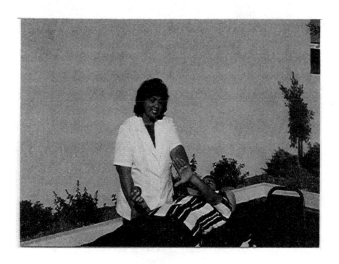

Figure 7-2
MRT with Allergen

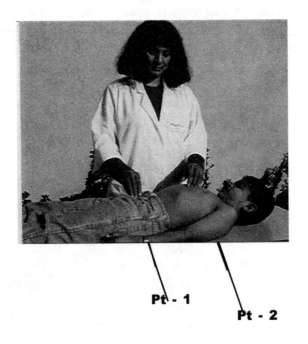

Pt - 1

Pt - 2

Figure 7-3
Balancing the Patient

by clearing the adverse energies of the allergens from the entire body. Thus it enables the body to relax, absorb and assimilate appropriate nutrients from the food that once caused allergies and support the proper growth of the entire body.

When some people are near allergens (adversely charged substances), they receive various clues from the brain, such as: an itchy throat, watery eyes, sneezing attacks, coughing spells, unexplained pain anywhere in the body, yawning, sudden tiredness, etc. You can demonstrate the changes in the weaknesses of the muscles by testing a strong indicator muscle in the absence of an allergen and then in its presence. The muscle will stay strong without any allergen in its electro-magnetic field, but will weaken in the presence of an allergen. This response of the muscle can be used to your advantage to demonstrate the presence of an allergen near you.

Muscle Response Testing

Muscle response testing can be performed in the following ways (See Illustrations of Muscle Response Testing on the Following Pages).

1. Standard muscle response test can be done in standing, sitting or lying positions. You need two people to do this test: the person who is testing, the "tester," and the person being tested, "the subject."

2. The "Oval Ring Test" can be used in testing yourself, and on a very a strong person with a strong arm. This requires only one person if you are self-testing. You need two people if you are testing another person.

3. Surrogate testing can be used in testing an infant, invalid person, extremely strong or very weak person, or an animal. The surrogate's muscle is tested by the tester, subject maintains skin-to-skin contact with the surrogate while being tested. The surro-

gate does not get affected by the testing. NAET treatments can also be administered through the surrogate very effectively without causing any interference with the surrogate's energy.

Two people are required to perform standard muscle response testing. The person who performs the test is called the tester, and the person who is being tested is called the subject. The subject can be tested lying down, standing or sitting. The lying-down position is the most convenient for both the tester and the subject; it also achieves more accurate results.

Step 1: The subject lies on a firm surface with one arm raised (left arm in the picture below) 90 degrees to the body with the palm facing outward and the thumb facing toward the big toe.

Step 2: The tester stands on the subject's (right) side. The subject's right arm is kept to his/her side with the palm either kept open to the air, or in a loose fist. The fingers should not touch any material, fabric or any part of the table the arm is resting on. This can give wrong test results. The left arm of the subject is raised 90 degrees to the body. The tester's left palm is contacting the subject's left wrist (Figure 7-1).

Step 3: The tester using the left arm tries to push down on the subject's raised left arm toward the subject's left big toe. The subject resists the push of the tester on the arm (the indicator muscle or pre-determined muscle). The PDM remains strong if the subject is well balanced at the time of testing. It is essential to test a strong PDM to get accurate results. If the muscle or raised arm is weak and gives way under pressure without the presence of an allergen, either the subject is not balanced, or the tester is performing the test improperly; For example, the tester might be trying to overpower the subject. The subject does not need to gather up strength from other muscles in the body to resist the tester with all his/her might. Only five to 10 pounds of pressure needs to be applied on the muscle for three to five seconds. If the muscle shows weakness, the tester will be able to judge the difference with only that small amount of pressure. Much practice is needed to test and sense the differences properly. If you cannot test properly or effectively the first few times, there is no need to get discouraged or frustrated. Please remember that practice makes you perfect.

Step 4: If the indicator muscle remains strong when tested a sign that the subject is found to be balanced - then the tester should put the suspected allergen into the palm of the subject's resting hand. The sensory receptors, on the tip of the fingers, are extremely sensitive in recognizing allergens. The fingertips have specialized sensory receptors that can send messages to and from the brain.

When the subject's fingertips touch the allergen, the sensory receptors sense the charges of the allergen and relay the message to the brain. If it is an incompatible charge, the strong PDM will go weak. If the charges are compatible to the body, the indicator muscle will remain strong. This way, you can test any number of items to determine the compatible and incompatible charges of the items against the body.

Step 5: This step is used if the patient is found to be out of balance as indicated by the indicator muscle or raised arm presenting weak— without the presence of an allergen. The tester then places his or her fingertips of one hand at 'point 1' on the mid-line of the subject, about one and a half inches below the navel. The other hand is placed on 'point 2', in the center of the chest on the mid-line, level with the nipple line. The tester taps these two points or massages gently clockwise with the fingertips about 20 or 30 seconds, then repeats steps 2 and 3. If the indicator muscle tests strong, continue on to step 4. If the indicator muscle tests weak again, repeat this process. Continue this procedure several times. It is very unlikely that any person will remain weak after repeating this procedure two to three times.

Point 1:

Name of the point: **Sea Of Energy**

Location: One and a half inches below the navel, on the midline.

This is where the energy of the body is stored in abundance. When the body senses any danger around its energy field or when the body experiences energy blockages, the energy supply is cut short and stored here. If you tap or massage clockwise on that energy reservoir point, the energy starts bubbling up and emerges from this point.

Point 2:

Name of the point: **Energy Distributor.**

Location: In the center of the chest on the midline of the body, level with the fourth intercostal space. This is the energy dispenser unit. From this center, energy is distributed to different tissues and organs as needed. This is the point that controls and regulates the energy circulation or Chi, in the body. When the energy rises from the Sea of Energy, it goes straight to the Energy Distributor point. From here, the energy is dispersed to different meridians, organs, tissues and cells as needed to help remove the energy blockages. It does this by forcing energy circulation from inside out. During this forced energy circulation, the blockages are pushed out of the body, balancing the body's state. You sense this through the strength of the indicator muscle.

The "Oval Ring Test" or "O Ring Test" can be used in self-testing, since this requires one person to perform the test. This can also be used to test a subject, if the subject is physically very strong with a strong arm and the tester is a physically weak person.

Step 1: The tester makes an "O" shape by opposing the little finger and thumb on the same hand. Then, with the index finger of the other hand he/she tries to separate the "O" ring against pres-

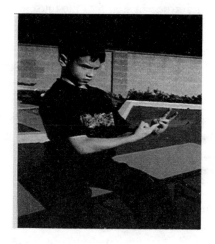

Self Testing

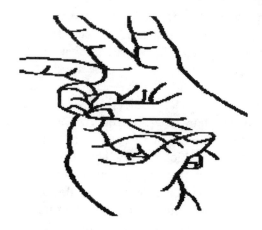

FIgure 7-4
`O' Ring Test to Detect Allergies

sure. If the ring separates easily, you need to use the balancing techniques as described in step 5 of the muscle response test.

Step 2: If the "O" ring remains inseparable and strong, hold the allergen in the other hand, by the fingertips, and perform step 1 again. If the "O" ring separates easily, the person is allergic to the substance he/she is touching. If the "O" ring remains strong, the substance is not an allergen. Muscle response testing is one of the most reliable methods of allergy tests, and it is fairly easy to learn and practice in every day life. This method cuts out expensive laboratory work.

After considerable practice, some people are able to test themselves very efficiently using these methods. It is very important for allergic people to learn some form of self-testing technique to screen out contact with possible allergens to prevent allergic reactions in order to have freedom to live in this chemically polluted world. After receiving the basic 30-40 treatments from a NAET practitioner, you will be free to live wherever you like if you know how to test and avoid unexpected allergens from your surroundings. Hundreds of new allergens are thrown into the world daily by non-allergic people who do not understand the predicament of allergic people. If you want to live in this world looking and feeling normal among normal people, side by side with the allergens, you need to learn how to test on your own. It is not practical for people to treat thousands of allergens from their surroundings or go to an NAET practitioner every day for the rest of their lives. You will not be free from allergies until you learn to test accurately. It takes many hours of practice. But do not get discouraged. I have given enough information on testing methods here. You have to spend time and practice until you reach perfection.

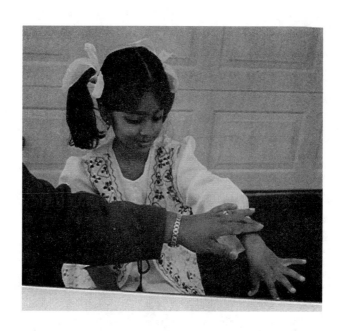

Figure 7-5
MRT in Sitting or Standing Position

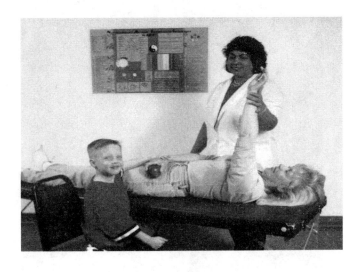

Figure 7-6
Surrogate Testing

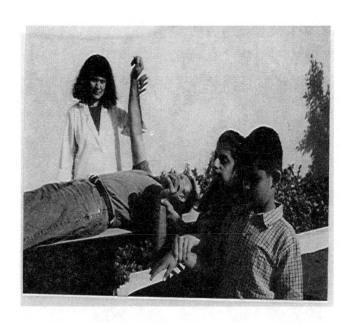

Figure 7-7
Extended Surrogate Testing

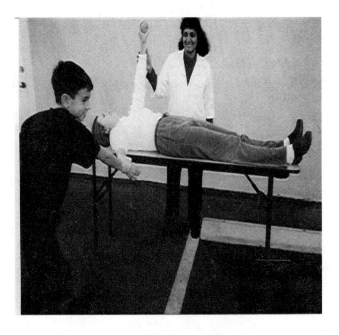

Figure 7-8
Testing a Hyperactive Child

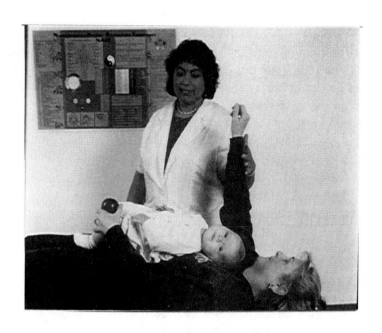

**Figure 7-9
Testing an Infant
Through a Surrogate**

A Tip to Master Self-testing

Find two items, one that you are allergic to and another that you are not, for example an apple and a banana.

You are allergic to the apple and not allergic to the banana. Hold the apple in the right hand and do the "Oval Ring Test" using your left hand. The ring easily breaks. The first few times if it didn't break, make it happen intentionally. Now hold the banana and do the same test. This time the ring doesn't break. Put the banana down, rub your hands together for 30 seconds. Take the apple and repeat the testing. Practice this every day until you can sense the difference. When you can feel the difference with these two items you can test anything around you.

Surrogate Testing

This method can be very useful to test and determine the allergies of an infant, a child, a hyperactive child, an autistic child, disabled person, an unconscious person, an extremely strong, and a very weak person, because they do not have enough muscle strength to perform an allergy test. You can also use this method to test an animal, plant, and a tree.

An extended surrogate testing is used when the patient (a hyperactive, an autistic, frightened child), is uncooperative. Three people are needed for this test as shown in Figure 7-7. NAET treatments can also be administered through the extended surrogate very effectively without causing any interference to the surrogate's energy.

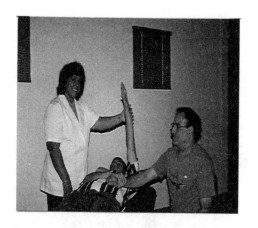

Figure 7-10
Testing To See If The Son
Is Allergic To The Father

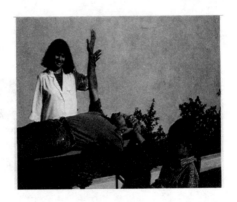

Figure 7-11
Testing to See if the Father
is Allergic to the Son.

The surrogate's muscle is tested by the tester. It is very important to remember to maintain skin-to-skin contact between the surrogate and the subject during the procedure. If you do not, then the surrogate will receive the results of testing and treatment.

NAET treatments can also be administered through the surrogate very effectively without causing any interference to the surrogate's energy. The testing or treatment does not affect surrogate as long as the subject maintains uninterrupted skin-to-skin contact with the surrogate.

As mentioned earlier, muscle response testing is one of the tools used by kinesiologists. Practiced in this country since 1964, it was originated by Dr. George Goodheart and his associates. Dr. John F. Thie advocates this method through the "Touch For Health" Foundation in Malibu, California. For more information and books available on the subject; interested readers can write to "Touch For Health" Foundation.

Muscle response testing can be used to test any substance for allergies. Even human beings can be tested for each other in this manner. When you are allergic to another human (father, mother, son, daughter, grandfather, grandmother, caretaker, baby sitter, etc.) you or your child could experience similar symptoms as you would with foods, chemicals or materials, whenever you or your child spends some time with the allergic person.

The subject lies down and touches the other person he or she wants tested (Figure 7-10, 7-11). The tester pushes the arm of the subject as in steps 2 and 3. If the subject is allergic to the second person, the indicator muscle goes weak. If the subject is not allergic, the indicator muscle remains strong.

If people are allergic to each other, (husband and wife, mother and child, father and son, patient and doctor, etc.) the allergy can affect a person in various ways. If the father and/or mother is allergic to the child, or child allergic to a parent or parents, child can get sick or remain sick indefinitely. The same things can happen to the parents too. If the husband is allergic to the wife or wife towards the husband, they can be fighting all the time and/or their health can be affected. The same things can happen among other family members too. It is important to test the family members and other immediate associates with your child for possible allergy and if found, they should be treated for each other to obtain good health and happiness.

Muscle response testing for allergies should be taught in every school and in every establishment. Everyone should learn to test to detect their allergies even if the treatment is not available. If you know your allergies, you can easily avoid them and that will help you somewhat.

Let's look at the history of 6-year-old Dominic who suffered from severe autism for 4 years. His mother Debbie brought Dominic to the office regularly for treatments. Before the treatment, he was spitting up every meal whether it was water or milk. He suffered from severe constipation, insomnia, irritability, colic pains and severe crying spells. He could not talk or communicate in words about his discomfort. Debbie spent extra time in the office to learn about autism and the NAET connection. She also took a special interest in the series of patient education seminars given in our office to the new patients once a week. Through the patient education seminars she learned ways to detect Dominic's untreated allergens before he was exposed to them. This made their lives easier.

She and her husband tested every food before they bought it from the store. Whenever they found an allergen, they avoided it until they brought the child to treat it with NAET. This helped Dominic immensely. He stopped having skin rashes and hives. He did not have too many temper tantrums any more. He slept well without nightmares and crying spells. Soon after Dominic received about 15-20 treatments, his disposition changed. He started talking, became friendlier, and his behavior changed. He was admitted to regular school. His mother became a teacher's assistant in his class so that she could keep a close watch on him. His parents continued to test him for everything before they introduced anything new to him. His parents took special care to feed him allergy-tested, or non-allergic food items only so that he could continue normal activities without interruption. Because of his mother's special attention, Dominic responded well to the treatment faster than any other autistic child I have ever treated before and he was able to have a normal school life. He is a healthy, intelligent ten-year-old now.

Just by knowing MRT and the testing procedure, Dominic's mother could prevent unwanted visits to the doctor's office. If we can teach these simple testing skills to all the parents of autistic children, the special education teachers, and the caretakers, and encourage them to use non-allergic products in the house, schools, and work-place, most allergy related autism could be controlled easily and these children could have a future like all other normal children.

Medical professionals as well as the public should be educated to listen and look for various types of allergies causing problem in various ways to all. Parents should form support groups to encourage other parents to learn MRT testing. Your normal children should be educated in testing. Schools should begin teaching muscle testing procedures to the children as a normal learning curriculum. Community centers, adult schools, hospitals involved in patient education sessions should take interest to teach MRT to all their attendees.

Allergies and allergy-related problems are on the rise due to our scientific advancements. If we learn to manage our adverse reactions towards the scientific advancements, we can enjoy the benefit of the modern inventions too. Unless you are educated to know about the MRT testing, you do not know what to look for. As you have seen, the theory of energy blockages and diseases comes from oriental medicine. Oriental medicine also teaches that, if given a chance, with a little support, the body will heal itself.

CHAPTER 8

BRAIN-BODY-LINKS

8

BRAIN-BODY-LINKS

The human body is made up of bones, flesh, nerves and blood vessels, which can only function in the presence of vital energy. Without this energy, the body is like an advanced efficient computer without an electrical power supply. Vital energy is not visible to the human eye, neither is electricity. No one knows how or why the vital energy gets into the body or how, when or where it goes when it leaves. However, it is true that without vital energy none of the body functions can take place. When the human body is alive vital energy flows freely through the energy pathways, the

---

blood will be circulating through the blood vessels and distributing appropriate nutrients to various parts of the body.

The blood helps to exchange oxygen and carbon dioxide cleaning up the impurities of the body. When blood receives proper nutrients, the body and bones grow, and the flesh and nerves, in turn, can protect the body; all body parts will work as a unit, like an efficient factory with all functions working as designed. When vital energy stops flowing through the energy pathways, the human machine ceases to function and the person is pronounced dead.

The human body is the most efficient, well-organized, functional unit known. Many branches of channels and energy pathways connect each and every cell of the body (the basic building block) with every other cell. In turn, every body part is connected and interlinked by a meshing networks of channels and branches, creating a perfect communication system within the body. The brain is the commander of this system. When the vital energy activates this system, the brain takes over the responsibilities. Under the brain's command, all parts of the body are activated; there is open communication between the brain, cells from different parts of tissue and other body parts. This communication takes place in a matter of nanoseconds; thus the brain maintains complete control of the body functions.

If for some reason a blockage takes place in the energy pathways, normal physiology is disrupted. This energy disruption will lead to certain visible effects in the human body and pathological symptoms will begin to appear. In the beginning, these pathological symptoms are seen around the blockage(s). Then they spread along the channels and branches to related tissues and organs. If the blockages affect the nerves that supply the different parts of the brain, diminished function of the brain is the result.

Traditional Chinese medicine describes the meridians as well as the symptoms of each of the primary channels. This chapter will explain the 12 primary channels and how blockages in these channels present physical and emotional symptoms, which cause illness, disease, and mental disorders. Many of the symptoms relating to blockages in the meridians will be familiar to the parents of children with autism. Only a brief overview is given in this chapter to aquaint you with energy meridians. You are encouraged to read or refer to any of the respective acupuncture textbooks named in the bibliography. Please read "Say Good-bye To Illness," by the author, for more extensive information about these meridians.

Lung Meridian

The inability of the lung meridian to accept fresh energy at 3:00 a.m. causes problems in the lung energy meridian. This blockage in the first meridian transmits into all other meridians as a chain reaction, and energy circulation gets disrupted.

Pathological Symptoms

• Afternoon fever, acute bronchial asthmatic attacks, asthma worse after 3:00 a.m., shortness of breath, burning in the eyes and nostrils, chest congestion, cough, coughing up blood, dry mouth and throat, emaciated look, fever, itching of the nostrils, headaches between eyes, nasal congestion, nose bleed, postnasal drips, runny nose with clear discharge, red or painful eyes, sneezing, throat irritation, swollen throat, and swollen cervical glands.

• Excessive perspiration in some cases and lack of perspiration in others, husky voice, infection in the respiratory tract, influenza, irritability, low voice, lack of desire to talk, laryngitis, nasal polyps, night sweats, other chest infections, pleurisy, pneumonia, red cheeks, red eyes, pain in the eyes, sinus infections, and sinus headaches.

• Abdominal bloating, nausea, vomiting, constipation or loose stools, body ache, irritability, and restlessness.

• Chronic hives, cradle cap, eczema, excessive sweating, skin rashes, skin tags, moles, warts, scaly and rough skin, heat sensation with hot palms, hair loss, thinning of the hair, poor growth of hair and nails, rough ridges on the nails, and brittle nails.

• Liking onion, peppers, garlic and cinnamon, pungent and spicy foods, and sometimes craving them.

Main Emotion : Grief

• Related emotions: a tendency toward humiliating others, always apologizing, comparing self with others, contempt, dejection, depression (early morning), despair, emotionally super sensitive, expressions of over-sympathy, false pride, low self-esteem, hopelessness, insulting others, and intolerance.

• Loneliness, meanness, melancholy, over demanding, prejudice, seeking others' approval, self-pity and weeping frequently without reason.

Essential Nutrition

Clear water, proteins, citrus fruits, cinnamon, onions, garlic, green peppers, black peppers, rice, vitamin C, bioflavonoids, and vitamin B-2.

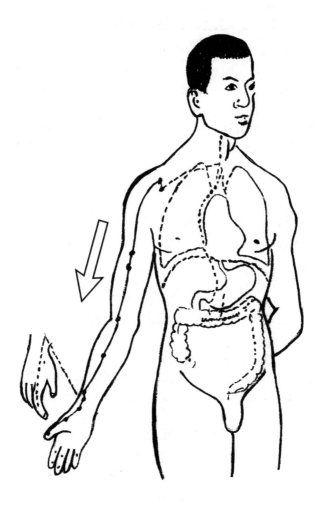

Figure 8-1
Lung Meridian (LU)

Large Intestine Meridian

Pathological Symptoms

- Dry mouth, dryness of the throat, sore throat, nose bleed, toothache on lateral incisors, first lower and second lower bicuspid, red and painful eyes, swelling of the neck and swelling of the lateral part of the knee joint, pain in the shoulders, knees, parts of the thighs, and along the course of the meridan.
- Lower abdominal cramps, constipation or diarrhea, spastic colon, spasms of the rectum and anal sphincter, itching of the anus, generalized hives, intestinal noise, flatulence, bleeding from the rectum, colitis, and dizziness.
- Abdominal pain, bloating, bad breath, belching, chest congestion, shortness of breath and sinus troubles and aches on the sides of the nose, between the eyes, and over the eyes.
- Acne, blister/inflammation of the lower gum, dermatitis, feeling better or tired after a bowel movement, hair loss, hair thinning, hives, and warts.

Main Emotion: Guilt

- Related Emotions: Grief, sadness, seeking sympathy, weeping, crying spells, and defensiveness.
- Haunted by past painful memories, bad dreams, nightmares, talking in the sleep, rolling restlessly in sleep, and inability to recall dreams.

Essential Nutrition

Vitamins A, D, E, C, B complex, especially B-1, wheat bran, oat bran, yogurt, and roughage.

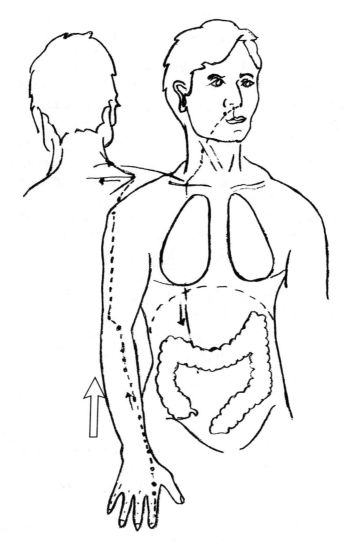

Figure 8-2
Large Intestine Meridian (LI)

Stomach Meridian

Pathological Symptoms

• Frequent fever, sore throat, coated tongue, flushed face, fever blisters, herpes, sores on the gums and inside the lips, red painful boils on the face, sweating, cracks on the center of the tongue, bad breath, fatigue, insomnia, seizures, toothache, pain on the upper jaw and upper gum diseases, fibromyalgia and temporo-mandibular joint problems (TMJ).

• Pain in the eye and chest, pain along the course of the channel in the leg or foot, swelling on the neck, facial paralysis, and coldness in the lower limbs.

• Acne, heat boils or blemishes, black and blue discoloration along the channel, itching and red rashes along the lateral aspect of the lower leg below the knee.

• Abdominal bloating, fullness or edema, abdominal cramps, vomiting, nausea, anorexia, bulimia, hiatal hernia, and discomfort when reclining.

• Insomnia, restlessness, mental confusion, personality changes, double personality, hyperactivity in children or adults, manic-depressive behaviors, learning disorders, schizophrenia, lack of concentration, and aggressive behaviors.

• Obsession, obsessive compulsive behaviors, panic disorders, headaches on the forehead, and behind the eyes (dull, sharp, pressure or burning pain behind the eyes).

Main Emotion: Disgust

• Related emotions: bitterness, disappointment, greed, emptiness, deprivation, restlessness, obsession, egotism,

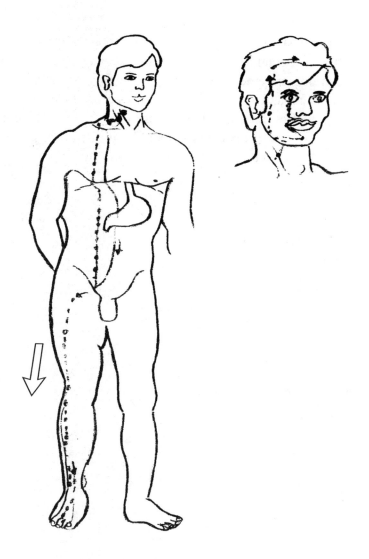

Figure 8-3
Stomach Meridian

and despair. Lack of concentration, nostalgia, mental confusion, mental fog, manic disorders, schizophrenia, hyperactivity, extreme nervousness, butterfly sensation in the stomach, and aggressive behaviors, paranoia, fear of losing control, fear of dying, terror (a sense that something unimaginably horrible is about to occur and one is powerless to prevent it), and perceptual distortions.

Essential Nutrition

B complex especially B-12, B-6, B-3 and folic acid and plenty of water.

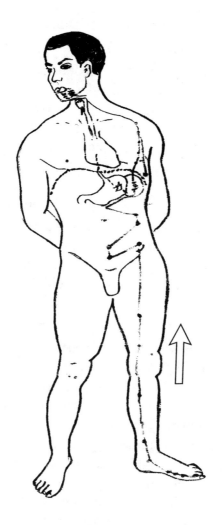

Figure 8-4
Spleen Meridian

Spleen Meridian

Pathological Symptoms

• Heaviness in the head, abdominal pain, fullness or distension, incomplete digestion of food, intestinal noises, nausea, vomiting, lack of taste, stiffness of the tongue, lack of smell, hard lumps in the abdomen, reduced appetite, craving sugar, loose stools, diarrhea, constipation, hypoglycemic reaction, general feverishness, and body aches.

• Low self-esteem, procrastination, depression, and intuitive and prophetic behaviors. Pallor, sleepy in the afternoon, latent insomnia, dreams that makes you tired, light-headedness, jaundice, fatigue, weak limbs, anemia, bleeding disorders, and hemorrhoids.

Main Emotion: Worry

• Related Emotions: Over-concern, nervousness, keeps feelings inside, likes loneliness, hyperactivity in children or adults, manic depressive disorder, obsessive compulsive disorder, panic attack, enjoy talking to self, and does not like crowds.

• Lack of self-confidence, gives more importance to self, hopelessness, irritable, likes to take revenge, likes to be praised, unable to make decisions, shy, timid, restrained, easily hurt, likes to get constant encouragement, otherwise falls apart, likes to live through others, over-sympathetic to others.

Essential Nutrition

Vitamin A, vitamin C, calcium, chromium, and protein.

Heart Meridian

Pathological Symptoms

This is one of the meridians often seen unbalanced in children with hyperactivity.

• Poor circulation and dizziness, general feverishness, headache, and dry throat.

• Mental disorders, nervousness, hyperactivity in children or adults, bipolar disorder, manic depressive disorder, depression, panic attack, obsessive compulsive disorder, emotional excesses, sometimes abusive, and irritability.

• Vertigo, nausea, dizziness, or light-headedness.

• Shortness of breath, excessive perspiration, insomnia, chest distension, palpitation, heaviness in the chest and sharp chest pain, irregular heart beats, and chest distention.

Main Emotion: Joy

• Over-excitement, emotional excess (excessive laughing or crying), sadness or lack of emotions.

• Abusive nature, bad manners, anger, easily upset, aggressive personality, insecurity, hostility, guilt, does not make friends, and does not trust anyone.

Essential Nutrition

Calcium, vitamin C, vitamin E, fatty acids, B complex and plenty of water.

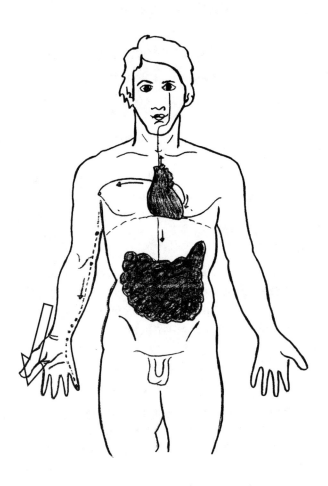

Figure 8-5
Heart Meridian

Small Intestine Meridian

Pathological Symptoms

- Distension and pain in the lower abdomen, pain radiating around the waist, and to the genitals.
- Abdominal pain with dry stool, constipation, and diarrhea. Knee pain, shoulder pain and frozen shoulder.

Main Emotion: Insecurity

- Related emotion: emotional instability, feeling of abandonment, or desertion.
- Joy, over-excitement, sadness, sorrow, and suppression of deep sorrow.
- Absent-mindedness, poor concentration, daydreaming paranoia, and sighing.
- Irritability, easily annoyed, lacking the confidence to assert oneself, and shy.
- Becoming too involved with details, introverted, and easily hurt.

Essential Nutrition

Vitamin B complex, vitamin D, vitamin E.
Acidophilus, yogurt, fibers, wheat germ, and whole grains.

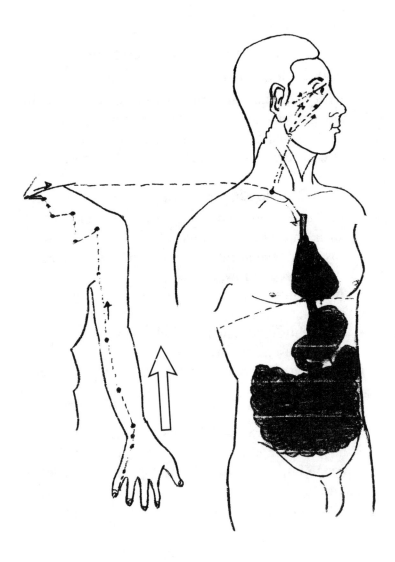

Figure 8-6
Small Intestine Meridian

Bladder Meridian

Pathological Symptoms

- Frequent, painful and burning urination, loss of bladder control and bloody urine.
- Chills, fever, headaches (especially at the back of the neck), stiff neck, nasal congestion, and disease of the eye.
- Pain: in the lower back, along back of the leg and foot, along the meridian, in the lateral part of the ankle, in the lateral part of the sole, in the little toe, and be hind the knee.
- Pain and discomfort in the lower abdomen, sciatic neuralgia, spasm behind the knee, spasms of the calf muscles, weakness in the rectum and rectal muscle.
- Pain in the lower abdomen, enuresis, retention of urine, burning urination, bloody urine, painful urination, frequent bladder infection, fever, and mental disorders.
- Chronic headaches at the back of the neck and pain at the inner canthus of the eyes.

Main Emotion: Fright

Related emotions: holds on to sad, disturbing and im pure thoughts, unable to let go of unwanted past memories, timid, inefficient, annoyed, highly irritable, fearful, unhappy, reluctant, restless, impatient, and frustrated.

Essential Nutrition

Vitamin C, A, E, B complex, B-1, calcium, and trace minerals.

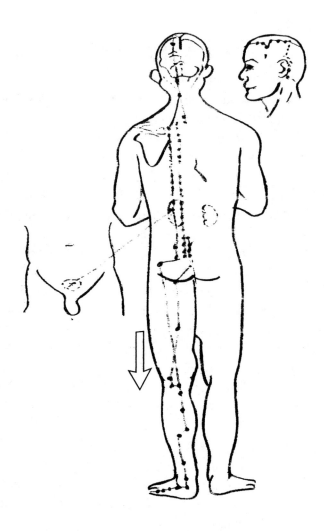

Figure 8-7
Bladder Meridian

KIDNEY MERIDIAN

Pathological Symptoms

- Pain: along the lower vertebrae, in the low back, and
- in the sole of the foot.
- Puffy eyes, bags under the eyes, and dark circles un der the eyes.
- Motor impairment or muscular atrophy of the foot, dryness of the mouth, sore throat, pain in the sole of the foot, pain in the posterior aspect of the leg or thigh, and lower backache.
- Pain and ringing in the ears, light-headedness, and nausea.
- Frequent burning, scanty and painful urination.
- Fever, fever with chills, irritability, vertigo, facial edema, blurred vision, ringing in the ears, spasms of the ankle and feet, swelling in the legs, and swollen ankles.
- Loose stools, chronic diarrhea, constipation, abdominal distention, vomiting, tiredness, dry mouth, excessive thirst, poor appetite, and poor memory.

Main Emotion: Fear

Related emotions: Indecision, terror, caution, confusion, seeks attention, unable to express feelings, lack of con centration, and poor memory.

Essential Nutrition

Vitamin A, E, B, essential fatty acids, calcium, and iron.

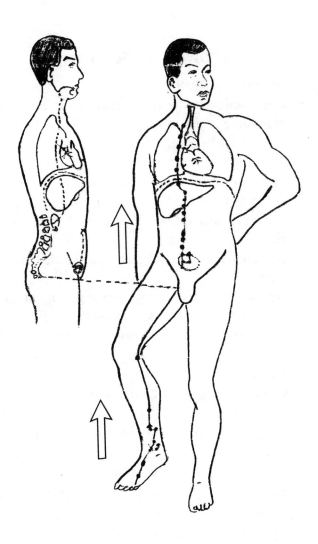

Figure 8-8
Kidney Meridian

PERICARDIUM MERIDIAN

Pathological Symptoms

- Stiff neck, spasms in the arm, in the leg, spasms of the elbow and arm, frozen shoulder, restricting movements hot palms, and pain along the channels.
- Impaired speech, fainting spells, flushed face, irritability, fullness in the chest, heaviness in the chest, slurred speech.
- Sensation of hot or cold, nausea, nervousness, pain in the eyes, and sub-axillary swellings.
- Motor impairment of the tongue, heaviness, palpitation and pain in the chest due to emotional overload.
- Irritability, excessive appetite, fullness in the chest, and sugar imbalance.

Main Emotion: Hurt or Joy

Related emotions: over-excitement, regret, jealousy, sexual tension, stubbornness, manic disorders, heaviness in the head, light sleep with dreams, fear of heights, various phobias, imbalance in sexual energy like never having enough sex or in some cases no sexual desire.

Essential Nutrition

Vitamin E, vitamin C, chromium, and trace minerals.

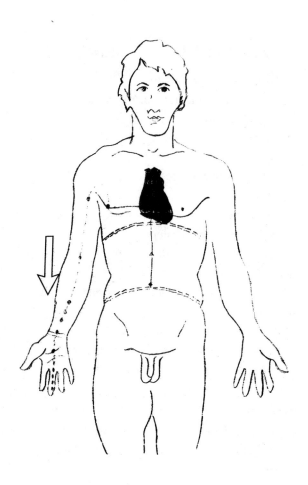

Figure 8-9
Pericardium Channel

Triple Warmer Meridian
Pathological Symptoms

- Swelling and pain in the throat, pain in the cheek and jaw, excessive hunger, redness in the eye, deafness, and pain behind the ear.

- Abdominal pain, distention, hardness and fullness in the lower abdomen, enuresis, frequent urination, and edema.

- Dysuria, excessive thirst, excessive hunger, always feels hungry even after eating, vertigo, indigestion, hypoglycemia, hyperglycemia, and constipation.

- Pain in the medial part of the knee, shoulder pain, and fever in the late evening.

Main Emotion: Hopelessness

Related emotions: depression, despair, grief, excessive emotion, emptiness, deprivation, and phobias.

Essential Nutrition

Iodine, table salt, trace minerals, vitamin C, calcium, fluoride, and water.

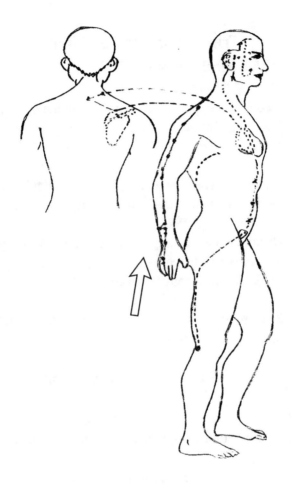

Figure 8-10
Triple Warmer Meridian

Gall Bladder Meridian

Pathological Symptoms

This meridian is unbalanced in people with autism.

• Alternating fever and chills, headache, ashen complexion, pain in the eye or jaw, swelling in subaxillary region, scrofula, and deafness.

• Pain along the channel in the hip region, leg or foot and along the channel, tremors or twitching of the body or parts of the body.

• Vomiting and bitter taste in the mouth, ashen complexion, swelling in the sub-axillary region and deafness.

• A heavy sensation in the right upper part of the abdomen, sighing, dizziness, chills, fever, and yellowish complexion.

Main Emotion: Rage

Related Emotions: assertion, aggression, shouting, and talking aloud.

Essential Nutrition

Vitamin A, calcium, linoleic acids, and oleic acids (for example, pine nuts).

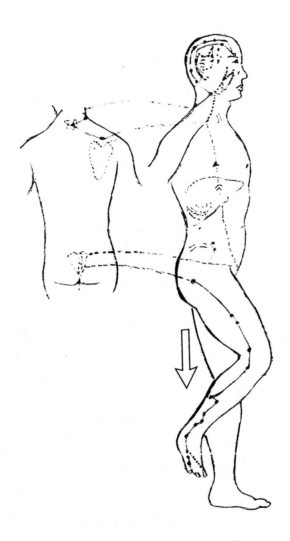

Figure 8-11
Gall Bladder Meridian

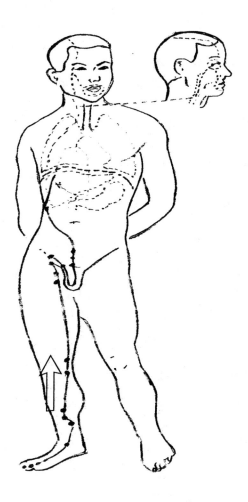

**Figure 8-12
Liver Meridian**

Liver Meridian

Pathological Symptoms

This meridian is unbalanced in people with autism.

- Headache at the top of the head, vertigo, and blurred vision.
- Feeling of some obstruction in the throat, tinnitus, fever, spasms in the extremities, abdominal pain, and hard lumps in the upper abdomen.
- Pain in the intercostal region, hernia, PMS, pain in the breasts, vomiting, jaundice, loose stools, and pain in the lower abdomen.
- Irregular menses, reproductive organ disturbances, and excessive bright colored bleeding during menses.
- Enuresis, retention of urine, dark urine, dizziness, and stroke- like condition.

Main Emotion: Anger

Related emotions: aggression, hyperactivity, frustration, unhappiness, complaining all the time, and finding faults with others.

Essential Nutrition

Beets, green vegetables, vitamin A, trace minerals, and unsaturated fatty acids.

CHAPTER 9

ALLERGY SELF-HELP

9

ALLERGY SELF-HELP

Most of the acupuncture points used in eliminating the energy blockages lie near vital organs. The information about the treatment points and the techniques for needling the specific points to remove allergy are not described in this book. Each of these points is needled with special techniques, which are taught in acupuncture colleges. Teaching these techniques is beyond the scope of this book and has been intentionally excluded. Needling in these areas requires proper education and extensive practice. Improper needling can cause damage to vital organs and even greater damage to health, sometimes leading to fatal accidents.

There are thousands of doctors trained in NEAT treatment methods all over the country. Please visit our website "naet.com" to find a practitioner near you.

Information regarding a few important acupuncture points is discussed in this chapter. They can be used to help control autism at any age. It is not a cure. It is going to provide temporary relief from the symptoms.

In Chapter eight we learned about the twelve acupuncture meridians and their pathological symptoms when the energy circulation is blocked in those meridians (diagrams 8-1 to 8-12). In Chapter 7, "Muscle-Response Testing," we learned to detect the cause of energy blockages by testing via MRT for allergies. We also found that allergies may be the causative agents for energy blockages in particular meridians. We have learned to test and find the causes in general. Practice these testing techniques and make a habit of testing your child for everything before exposing yourself, or your child to food, clothing, household chemicals, drugs, immunizations and environmental agents, etc., which you know or suspect are allergens.

NAET SUPPLEMENTATION

This can also be used to test for adequate dosages of medications, too.

Find an indicator muscle. Have the patient hold one vitamin pill (e.g. calcium) in his/her free hand. Test the indicator muscle x 3. If weak, then the patient is allergic to the pill. Treat the patient for that pill using NAET.

If strong, add more pills to his/her hand, until his/her hand goes weak again.

Now, count the pills in his/her hand. The total number in his/her hand is his/her deficiency.

This number can be anywhere from 1-2 pills to many thousands in the case of vitamin deficiency.

If the deficiency is 1-6 pills, he/she may not need to take too many supplements. He/she can eat a balanced meal or take a one-a-day vitamin. If the deficiency is more than 6 pills (6x daily dosage) and under 10 pills, supplement 1 pill daily. If the deficiency is many tens, hundreds or thousands, then supplement 4-6 times normal daily doses a day until the deficiency is taken care of.

When there is no more deficiency in the patient, he/she can eat a balanced meal or take a one-a-day vitamin.

When the patient is not allergic toward a substance anymore, the body will naturally demonstrate a need for that item. Then you need to supplement adequately. If you depend to receive the nutrients from the food alone it may take a few years before your body can fill up the deficiency. Appropriate supplementation will help to bring the patient's body to a balance by alleviating the long-term deficiency that was caused by the allergy. It is essential to supplement the patient appropriately to achieve better and faster results when the allergy is successfully treated.

Acu points Massage to Balance A Child

Begin the day for a child with an acu-point massage. The acupoints are shown in the diagram Simply apply gentle finger pressure on the points in the order given in the diagram. Fifteen seconds on each point twice a day, in the morning when waking up and before going to sleep. Begin from point 1 in the diagram (9-1) and go in order to point 10 and finish up in the right hand at point-1. This will encourage the energy to move in the clockwise direction. When the energy circulates in the right direction, it will stabilize the body by bringing the body function into a homeostasis. The points are numbered in the right order of treatment for easy understanding. This can be used in balancing the energy in acute phase of a disease also. Whichever organ or meridian is causing problem (find that out by MRT), find the appropriate organ-meridian connecting point and apply gentle pressure at the point for a couple of minutes. This might bring relief in the particular organ and meridian.

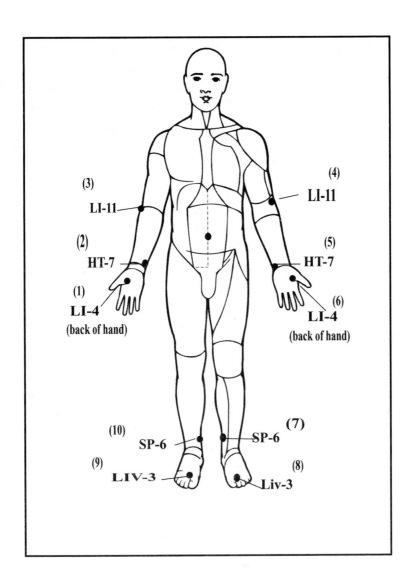

Figure: 9-1
General Balancing Points

Acu help Points

Find the appropriate point from diagram 9-2. Apply slight finger pressure, with the pad of your index finger, on the point. Hold 1-3 minutes at each point. Try to repeat the procedure three-four times a day. If your child is suffering from an acute attack, you may work with acuhelp points every five to ten minutes until the problems gets under control. Please learn the location from the diagram.

Location of Acu-help points.

GV-20: Center of the top of the head.

Lung -1: In the depression below the acromial extremity of the clavicle, 8 finger breadths lateral to the midline.

Thymus: beginning from the lower border of the supraclavicular fossa and extends to the upper border of the xyphoid process of the sternum.

LI-11: when the elbow is flexed, it is at the end of the elbow crease.

LI-4: midway between the thumb and index finger approximately one body inch above the web.

HT-7: medial side of the transverse crease of the wrist.

PC-6: three finger breadths above the wrist crease on the palmer side.

Lu-7: superior to the styloid process of the radius, two finger breadths above the transverse crease of the wrist.

CV-12:on the midline of the abdomen, 5 finger breadths above the navel.

SP-10: when the knee is flexed, 3 finger breadths above the superior border of the patella, on the medial side of the thigh.

ST-36: four finger breadths below the eye of the patella, one finger breadth lateral from the anterior crest of the tibia.

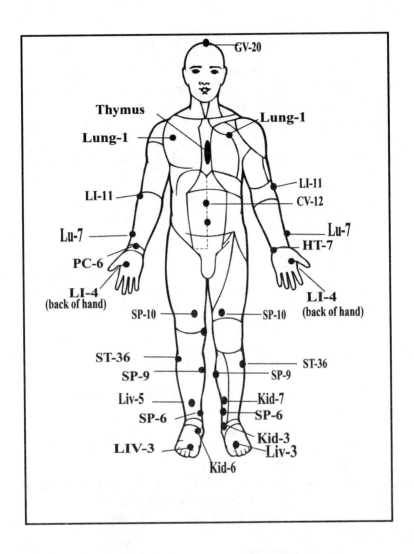

FIgure: 9-2
Acuhelp Points

SP-9: on the lower border of the medial condyle of the tibia in the depression between the posterior border of the tibia and gastrocnemius muscle.

SP-6: 4 finger breadths directly above the tip of the medial malleolus.

Liv-5: 7 finger breadths above the tip of the medial malleolus on the medial border of tibia.

Kid-7: 3 finger breadths directly above kidney-3, on the anterior border of the tendo-calcaneus.

Kid-3: in the depression between the medial malleolus and tendo-calcaneus, level with the tip of the medial malleolus.

Kid-6: two finger breadths below the medial malleolus.

Liv-3: in the depression distal to the junction on the 1st and 2nd metatarsal bones.

NAET Child-help

Find the allergen causing the immediate problem (asthma, shortness of breath, fever, seizures, etc.) by testing with MRT using the information from chapter 7.

Put the substance in a glass jar with a lid or a test tube.

Look at the diagram 9-3. Make the child lie on a flat surface (perhaps on a table). Support the child or hold the child with one hand over the clothes. Keep the allergen near the child in contact with the child's body. Gently stroke neck down as shown in the diagram for 13 strokes at a time, repeating the cycles every ten minutes until the child feels better.

After the acute phase, take the child to an NAET practitioner and get the NAET basic 25 treated. This will help to prevent future similar attacks.

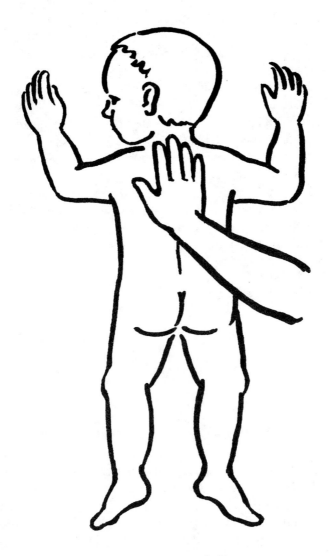

Figure: 9-3

NAET Child-help

Treating Patients with the History of Anaphylaxis

Always complete at least fifteen NAET basics before treating for severely allergic item. Always test the patient with the history of severe allergies through a surrogate. Do not let the patient touch the sample diectly. Have the sample in a glass jar and let the surrogate hold it in the opposite hand where the patient will have the contact. While checking for the weak areas, patient remains away from the hand of the surrogate where the sample is held. Treat the child through surrogate only. After the treatment, patient should not hold the sample for the usual 20 minutes. Follow rest of the instruction for the treatment as regular NAET protocol. Ask the patient to massage on the general balancing points every 2-4 hours during the 25 hours. On the next visit, check the item thoroughly for the organs, levels, and possible combinations and if needed treat for all the necessary combinations as many times as needed until the NAET doctor is satisfied with the result of the treatment. In some extremely severe cases, it has taken 10-15 treatments (one treatment per day) to eliminate an allergy to an item that has caused anaphylactic reactions in the past (some of the items treated successfully with NAET and now patients are using these products successfully are penicillin, aspirin, mushroom, shellfish, peanuts, milk, egg, iodine, hair dye, perfume, formaldehyde, and latex). After you are satisfied about the result, if you cannot find any more combinations, have the patient hold the item in a glass jar with a lid and make her sit in your office for half-an-hour every day for a week. After that let her touch the item in her hand without the glass jar, every day for half-hour to an hour for a week. If the patient does not show any more adverse symptoms with these contact, then on the next visit, he/she can put a portion of it in his/her mouth and wait for a few minutes, then spit it out and rinse the mouth with clear water, every day for a few days. If the patient did not have any reaction during this observation period, if patient wants to eat, he/she will be able to eat. In cases of peanut butter allergies, you don't have to make the child eat a peanut butter sandwich every day, but the treatment is mainly for preventing anaphylaxis and other unpleasant reactions when they are among other people eating around them.

The Cephalic Rub

According to Chinese medical principles, all Yang meridians pass through the head traveling close to the superficial level reporting each and every energetic activity of every instant to the brain. All Yin meridians also pass through the head at a deeper level supporting and confirming the finding of their counterparts, Yang meridians, according to *Tang Dynasty physician Sun Si-Mo, "The three hundred connecting channels all rise to the head."* When you massage the whole head gently with a kneading movement, you are in fact invigorating all the energy meridians forcing the energy blockages to come out of the meridians and helping the energy to circulate freely through the energy pathways. When the energy circulates freely, blood circulation improves by allowing the oxygen and nutrients to reach every part of the brain evenly.

If anyone experiences pain or other discomfort (seizure activities, etc.) you should consult your physician for assistance. Child may be harboring toxins in the upper part of the body mainly in the different lobes or parts of the brain (parietal lobe, frontal lobe, occipital lobe, temporal lobe, pons, midbrain, cerebellum, corpus callosum, etc.), and the massage invigorates the circulation in certain area of the brain, by assisting the toxin out of the trapped segment. Sometimes mild massage is not sufficient to bring the toxin out of its hiding place and may cause previous or existing symptoms to recur until the toxin is cleared completely. Commonly seen toxic symptoms are headaches, runny nose, watering of the

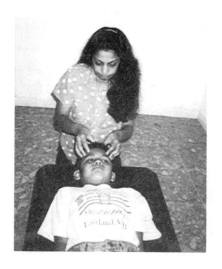

Figure: 9-4
Cephalic Rub

eyes, ear aches, mild seizures (if one already has the history of such symptoms in the past). Toxins may have accumulated from previous or recent reactions from bacterial infection, viral infection or parasites infestation, or heavy toxins from pesticides, heavy metals, mercury, etc., in the energy meridians. Such problems should be solved before proceding with energy invigorating treatments such as cephalic rub.

A-fifteen-minute massage, once every other day will help to nourish and stabilize the brain. After the head massage the person should lie down flat for an hour allowing the energy to concentrate in the brain tissues allowing enough time for the toxins to move into the blood or lymphatic circulation and to find it's way out of the body.. The best time to do this head massage is before bedtime.

Procedure

The massage can be done using any of the following items. You should make sure that the child is not allergic to the substance you are using for massage.

Massage oil
Olive oil
Coconut oil
Clarified butter
Grapeseed oil
Any other oil
Cooked mung bean paste
Buckwheat paste
Cooked brown rice paste

Cook brown rice or mung bean with the skin still on. After bringing it to room temperature blend it with a few drops of oil. Massage the whole head gently for 15 minutes with this nutrient paste once a week. Wait for 30 minutes to an hour, then wash the head thoroughly and dry it.

Pioneer medical experts believed massaging with nourishing nutrients would help to nourish the brain faster (allowing the nutrients to get into the system by osmosis?). Massaging once a week with any of these nutrients or in combination of multiple nutrients have produced good results in some cases.

Thymus Stimulation

Thymus gland stimulation helps to improve the immune system reducing the allergic reactions. Since children have poor immune systems and susceptible to get severe allergies, thymus stimulation has been very helpful in reducing allergies by improving their immune system.

Procedure

Make the child lie down in a comfortable place in supine position (lie on the back), preferably on the bed. A simple clockwise, gentle massage on the thymus gland for 1-3 minutee twice a day, preferably in the morning and before going to bed at night will nurture the thymus gland. For location of the area refer to Figure 9-5.

Meridian Balancing

Have a set of meridian therapy cards, an energy chart or look at the travel pathways of twelve acupuncture meridians in Chapter eight of this book or Chapter 10 in "Say Good-bye to Illness," by the author. Meridian therapy cards are available from the NAET website store: www.naet.com. Gently trace the meridians bilateral on your child's body from the beginning of the first

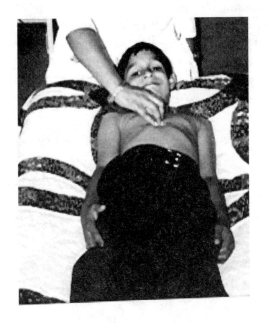

Figure: 9-5
Thymus Stimulation

meridian of the energy cycle (Lung meridian) to the last one (Liver meridian). Run your fingers over the meridians with a gentle stroking action toward their flow (marked with 'start' and 'end' in the beginning and end of the meridians and an arrow denoting the

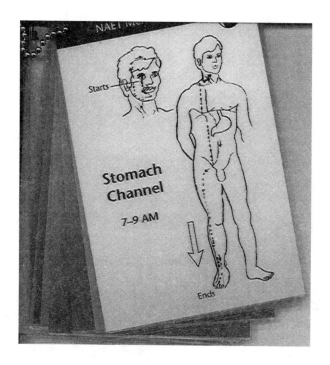

Figure: 9-6
Meridian Cards

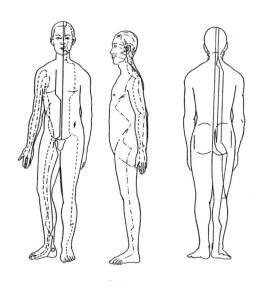

Figure: 9-7
Major Energy Meridians of the Body

Resuscitation Points

1. Fainting: GV 26, GB 12, LI 1, PC 9, KID 1
2. Nausea: CV 12, PC 6
3. Backache: GV 26, UB 40
4. Fatigue: CV 5, LI 1, CV 17
5. Fever: LI 11, LU 10, GV 16

For more information on revival techniques, refer to Chapter 3, pages 570 to 573, in "Acupuncture: A Comprehensive Text," by Shanghai College of Traditional Medicine, Eastland Press, 1981 or refer to "Living Pain Free with Acupressure" by the author. It is available at various bookstores and at our **website (naet.com).**

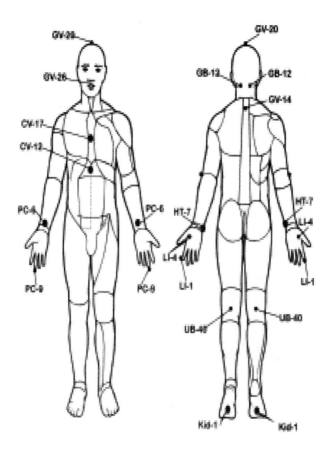

Figure 9-8
Resuscitation Points

Supplemental Procedures

Fresh leaves, flowers, buds, sprouts, seeds, essential oils, essence, roots and barks of the plants and trees have been used from the earliest civilization by men for some of these following purposes:

- to flavor the food and drinks
- to decorate the houses
- to protect the body from invaders (bacteria, parasites, etc.),
- to cleanse the inside and outside the body
- to treat various ailments and health disorders
- to beautify the body

Herbal drinks

Pour boiling water into a cup with a lid and add the appropriate herbal leaves, seeds, flowers, pollens, roots, powders, etc., let the herbs soak in the boiling water for three to five minutes. Strain and drink the tea as you need it. Add sugar, or honey to taste.

Anise	Ginger fresh or dried
Basil	Hibiscus
Baking soda	Honey
Black pepper	Jasmine
Butter	Lemon
Camelia	Lemon grass
Camphor	Lemon leaves
Chrisanthemum	Menthol
Cinnamon	Mint
Cloves	Nutmeg
Cumin	Olive
Garlic	Onion

Herbs with Healing Properties:

1. Steam Inhalation to Clear Respiratory Passages
Preparation:

Use this steam bath, inhalation or fomentation on grown up children (over ten years old). For small children use the second technique. In a large, heatproof bowl, pour steaming water. You can add leaves, flowers fresh or dried, seeds, pollens, barks, teabags, essential oils, essence, or tablets of the kind of herb you want to use. Add leaves, barks and seeds in the water and boil the water for 20 minutes. Add the flowers to the bowl when you pour the steaming water and keep it covered for 2 minutes before using the steam inhalation or bath. When you use oils or herbal essence let the water cool a little before adding the oil drops; otherwise the oils can evaporate quickly.

Create a tent by wrapping a bath towel around your head and drape it over the outer rim of the bowl. Sit with your face about 1 to 1 1/2 feet away from the bowl. Close your eyes and enjoy the relaxing steam. Take a few deep breaths. Try to inhale the steam through your nose and let it out through your mouth. Inhale the steam and allow the steam penetrate your nasal passages, face, neck for about 10 minutes if you can tolerate. 3-5 minutes will be okay too. Avoid scalding or burning. Never do this on small children under ten. Never leave children unattended.

You can also use vicks vaporub or tablet, lemon barks, mint leaves, menthol, or lemon rind, instead of lemon leaves.

Alternative Technique for
Little Children and Infants

For infants/ small children: Keep the pan with steaming water in the bath room and seat the child or infant a few feet away from the pan. Close all the doors and windows. Open the lid completely and let the steam spread in the room. Keep the child/infant 1 foot away from the pan for 20 minutes. The vapor in the room will be sufficient to humidify the infant's lungs to loosen up the phlegm. You can also run the hot water for ten minutes in the bathroom with closed doors and windows. Then bring the child/infant in and leave him/her for five to ten minutes in the bath room near the bowl with herbal water. This will help to fill up the room with steam faster.

How Does It Work?

Steam bath is used in humidifying the respiratory passages and sinuses, by stimulating the drainage of the mucus by opening up the clogged up mucus producing cells, sinuses and glands.

Indication: nasal congestion, shortness of breath due to common colds, influenza, reduce runny nose, cough and laryngitis followed by common colds. Herbs will work as therapeutic agents.

- Lemon leaves: good to stop cough by opening up the nasal passages, throat, and larynx and eliminating the phlegm.
- Cinnamon: Helps to improve the energy in weak children who are too weak to cough up the phlegm. This is also helpful to prevent bad smell from the nasal passages due to clogged up old yellow, thick, mucus.
- Fresh ginger: to reduce pain
- Menthol/vicks and mint : Good to reduce sore throat.
- Hibiscus: Eliminate toxins

Lemon grass: Helps with pain in the face and sinuses.

After the steam inhalation wrap the child (especially the chest and neck area) with a warm blanket or scarf for twenty minutes. Give a warm drink to sip on while sitting with the wrap.

Do it twice a day for a couple of days or more days if you need it.

Steam Fomentation For Skin

Do the same above procedure. Add 1/4 teaspoonful of turmeric powder, rose petals, hibiscus petals in the pan and let it sit for a few seconds. Open the lid of the pan and allow the heat flow on to your face and neck by controlling the tent over the bowl. Keep your face two feet away from the pan in order to prevent burns or scalding from the hot steam. This will open up the clogged up sebaceous glands and clean up the pores on the skin. Turmeric is also antibacterial and promote healing.

Used in: acne, eczema, dermatitis, itching of the skin on the face and facial pain.

Epsom Salt Bath

Epsom salt tub bath:

Fill up the bath tub with desired amount of lukewarm water. Add 1 cupful of Epsom salt into the water and dissolve it. Make the child sit in the bath tub and soak for 30 minute. Little children should not be left alone in the tub full of water.

Epsom salt sitz bath:

Fill up the bath tub with less water just to sit in the water. A plastic or metal bucket or pan with appropriate size can be used to soak different areas of the body (foot bath, hand bath, etc.).

Vinegar Bath

Vinegar bath:

Fill up the bath tub with desired amount of lukewarm water. Add 1 cupful of white vinegar into the water and stir it. Make the child sit in the bath tub and soak for 30 minute. Little children should not be left alone in the tub full of water.

Vinegar sitz bath:

Fill up the bath tub with less water just to sit in the water. A plastic or metal bucket or pan with appropriate size can be used to soak different areas of the body (foot bath, hand bath, etc.).

Vinegar bath is good for eczema, dermatitis, rough skin of the face, feet, hands, etc.

You may also substitute other leaves, flowers, oils, essences, extracts, powders, and herbal products in the bath same way. Different herbs are used for different purposes but preparation of teas and baths are done the same way.

It is a good idea to use a room humidifier.

CHAPTER 10

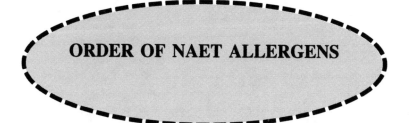

ORDER OF NAET ALLERGENS

10

ORDER OF NAET ALLERGENS

C hildren suffering from frequent everyday ailments are found to be allergic to many food and environmental substances. We have found most of these children are reactive to the commonly used everyday food items.

The following food groups are listed according to their importance for the body. It is necessary to avoid the allergen for 25 hours following the allergy elimination treatment. Please follow your NAET specialist's instructions carefully along with the diet during the 25 hours after the treatment in order to be free from the allergen successfully. On occasion, in certain cases it is possible to reduce the number of hours of avoidance. Your NAET doctor would test your child and inform you of the exact number of hours of avoidance necessary for the individual child after completion of each treatment before you leave the office. In children it is difficult to restrict the allergen for 25 hours as it is done on adults. When you avoid the allergen for limited hours only (instead of 25 hours) in some cases, it has been found that treatment for the particular item may need to be repeated either alone or by various different combinations in the future. Even if there is a possibility of future treatments on the item, most parents like to go for the short span of avoidance of 4-5 hours instead of 25 hours on children.

You may also refer to the NAET Guidebook for more information on NAET treatments and specific food to eat and instructions to follow during the avoidance period.

Most children can get their symptoms under control when they complete NAET group-A of allergens successfully. Some children with mild to moderate symptoms would show marked improvements after they complete just five basic groups of allergens. But it is to their advantage to complete the 15-40 groups of allergens before they stop the treatments.

1. Egg Mix (egg white, egg yolk, chicken, tetracycline and feathers).

You may eat brown or white rice, pasta without eggs, vegetables, fruits, milk products, oils, beef, pork, fish, coffee, juice, soft drinks, water, and tea.

Danny, 9-years-old, suffered from asthma, and eczema. His mother told us he was having difficulty reading in school and lacked energy. When he came home from school he always took a nap before he could do his homework. In our office we tested him through NTT and found that he was extremely allergic to eggs and chicken, which caused a severe energy blockage in his lungs (asthma), spleen (fatigue), and colon meridians (eczema). His mother told us that eggs and chicken were practically Danny's entire diet. He loved scrambled or hard boiled eggs for breakfast. Egg salad or chicken sandwiches were always in his lunch bag. On the weekends he would ask for omelettes or fried chicken. His favorite dessert was vanilla custard made with whole eggs. Checking further we found that he slept on feather pillows and had a down comforter. We told his mother to remove everything with feathers from Danny's room and take eggs and chicken out of his diet for a week. The following week they returned for the egg mix treatment. He needed to be treated separately for egg white, egg yolk, and chicken and tetracycline, before he cleared the treatment for egg mix. Danny's asthma, eczema and fatigue are no longer a problem. When I asked Danny how he was doing in school, the big smile on his face said it all.

2. Milk and Calcium (breast milk, cow's milk, goat's milk, casein, albumin, and calcium).

You may eat cooked rice, (no raw fruits or vegetables) cooked heated and cooled fruit juices, and vegetables (like potato, squash, green beans, yams, cauliflower, sweet potato), chicken, red meat, salt, oils, and drink calcium-free water, coffee and tea without milk.

Jimmy, 12-years-old, was not growing as fast as the other boys on his baseball team. He complained of leg cramps after baseball practice. His parents were concerned and saw a nutritionist. The nutritionist advised them to give Jimmy calcium supplements. Within one week of taking the supplements, he began to get severe joint pains and became sick. Jimmy was tested for calcium and found to be allergic to it. After treatment using NAET, his cramps and joint pains subsided. When he began taking calcium after clearing his allergy, he became stronger and grew several inches in a few months, catching up to the rest of his team.

An eighteen-month-old girl was brought to our clinic because she was having heart palpitations. She cried constantly after eating and her mother was a nervous wreck. Muscle testing using her mother as a surrogate, we found the little girl to be allergic to milk and milk products, which she was eating or drinking at every meal. After NAET treatment for calcium, her heart palpitations and constant crying stopped. Her heart palpitations haven't returned since. She now is a healthy five-year-old.

Three-month-old Katie had skin rashes all over her body. Her mother put gloves on her at night to keep her from scratching. Katie was always restless and it was difficult to get her to take a nap or go to sleep. After breast-feeding Katie would cry and cry. Katie slept calmly and her rashes disappeared after treatment for her mother's breast milk.

3. Vitamin C (fruits, vegetables, vinegar, citrus, bioflavonoids, rutin, berry, vitamin C, ascorbic acid, Oxalic acid, and citric acid).

You may eat cooked white or brown rice, pasta without sauce, boiled or poached eggs, baked or broiled chicken, fish, red meat, brown toast, deep fried food, French fries, salt, oils, and drink coffee or water.

An eight-year-old girl's throat would swell whenever she ran or participated in physical exercises at school or at home. Lately, just walking briskly would cause her throat to constrict. Her worried mother brought her to our clinic. She was keeping the girl at home because she was so frightened she would not be able to breathe if she participated in anything at school. Muscle testing showed her to be highly allergic to Vitamin C and citrus bioflavonoid. She loved fruits, especially oranges. Her mother always packed an orange in her lunch bag and she drank orange juice at recess, then played on the playground. After passing the treatment for Vitamin C and bioflavonoids she runs and jumps rope without any swelling in her throat.

4. B complex vitamins

You may only eat cooked white rice, cookies and bread or pancakes made with white flour, cauliflower raw or cooked, well cooked or deep fried fish, salt, white sugar just for taste in a limited amount (no brown sugar or natural syrups), black coffee, French fries, and purified water when treating for any of the B vitamins. Rice should be washed well before cooking. It should be cooked in lots of water and drained well to remove the fortified vitamins. Since sugar is a helper of B vitamins, consuming too much sugar or eating sugary foods during the 25 hour period following B vitamins can cause treatment failure.

When Jean, a patient of ours, came to our office she was tired and upset. Her daughter and newborn baby were visiting for two weeks and her little granddaughter had been crying constantly. Her daughter would hold the infant in her arms day and night, but she just cried and cried. They would take turns staying up at night She would cry during her bottle feeding, and would spit up much of her formula. Jean asked if she could bring her baby to the clinic for me to see. She returned the next day with her daughter and granddaughter. The baby was still crying. Her stomach was bloated and her mother said the baby was either constipated or had diarrhea. Muscle testing using her mother as a surrogate, we found that she was allergic to the baby formula she was drinking. We immediately treated her for the formula (using her mother as a surrogate). We had to treat her several times before she cleared for the baby formula. The crying stopped and her bowel movements returned to normal once she passed the treatment.

Another infant, 7-months-old, developed irritable bowel syndrome. He began losing weight and couldn't digest his food. We traced the problem to the introduction of cereals into his diet. Rice, wheat and corn were the culprits in his case. After being treated for the basic ten food groups, his irritable bowel symptoms disappeared.

5. Sugar Mix (cane sugar, corn sugar, maple sugar, grape sugar, rice sugar, brown sugar, beet sugar, fructose, molasses, honey, dextrose, glucose, and maltose).

You may eat white rice (white rice is pure starch, it is okay to eat since it takes time to convert into sugar; brown rice contains immediately available rice sugar in it), pasta, vegetables, vegetable oils, meats, eggs, chicken, water, coffee, tea without milk. Avoid fruits.

Todd, 6-years-old, was having difficulty in first grade. He couldn't get along with the other children, follow directions or wait his turn. Sitting still was impossible for him so he walked around the room or rolled on the floor. He wasn't able to read the simplest words or add numbers to ten. His teacher had told his mother that he really wasn't ready for first grade. His mother brought him to our clinic. Todd was an only child and his mother was very protective of him. She said he didn't behave badly at home, although he was restless and had a short attention span. We tested and found something Todd was eating was causing his behavioral problems. His mother said she only gave him healthy foods, never refined or processed products to eat. Checking through muscle testing, we found he was allergic to sugar. His mother was certain she never gave him sugar. When she made him desserts or cookies she always sweetened them with *honey or molasses. I explained to her that honey and molasses work the same way refined sugar does in the body. After treating Todd for Sugar Mix, his behavior improved dramatically. He could sit still in class. He began to read and his addition was perfect. He is doing well in school now and even eating cookies made with refined sugar without any of his previous symptoms.*

6. Iron Mix (animal and vegetable sources: beef, pork, lamb, raisin, date, seeds, nuts, and broccoli).

You may eat white rice without iron fortification, sourdough bread without iron, cauliflower, white potato, chicken, light green vegetables (white cabbage, iceberg lettuce, white squash), yellow squash, and orange juice.

Cindy was a very active teenager. She was a cheerleader, played the flute and was on the track team at her junior high school. When she turned fourteen she began experiencing back-aches. Sometimes they were so severe she missed school. She had to give up cheerleading and became an alternate on the track team. Her mother took her to the family doctor who had ordered a blood test. Cindy was found to be anemic. The doctor prescribed iron tablets and told her to get some bed rest for her back. Instead of improving, her symptoms became more severe. A neighbor, a patient of mine, recommended that she make an appointment to see me. Cindy was in severe pain on her first visit to the clinic. It was difficult for her to sit in one position for a long period of time. After testing her we found that she was allergic to bananas, peaches, apricots, raisins, cereals, beans, red meats, spinach, egg yolk, clams and oysters. All these foods had one thing in common: they contained iron. She began the basic ten treatments. After passing the treatment for iron, and supplementing with iron, she no longer was anemic and her backaches disappeared. She was able to be back on the track team and was jumping up and down as a cheerleader again.

7. Vitamin A (animal and vegetable source, beta carotene, fish and shell fish).

You may eat cooked white rice, products made from white flour, pasta, potato, cauliflower, red apples, chicken, water, and coffee.

Greg, ten-years-old, would wake up with mild headaches. By afternoon the pain would be so severe that it interfered with his schoolwork. He would become agitated and angry with his classmates. He rarely paid attention in class. After a parent conference, his mother took Greg to the doctor. He was diagnosed as having migraines and given medication to control pain.

He was still having migraines when he came to our office. He told us his headaches would get really painful late morning and continued throughout the afternoon. I asked Greg to tell me what he usually ate during the day. The only food that he ate on a regular basis was carrot sticks. He would have them for his snack everyday at recess. Sometimes he ate more carrot sticks at lunch. He was tested for Vitamin A and was allergic to it. The day after the treatment, Greg ran in to my office to tell me the good news. He didn't have a trace of a headache all day. The carrots were the cause of his allergy induced headaches.

8. Mineral Mix (magnesium, manganese, phosphorus, selenium, zinc, copper, cobalt, chromium, trace minerals, gold, and fluoride).

You may use only distilled water for washing, drinking, and showering. You may eat cooked rice, vegetables, fruits, meats, eggs, salt, oils, and drink milk, coffee, tea and distilled water. Avoid root vegetables (onions, potato, etc.).

Seven-year-old Danny was having frequent asthma attacks that were so severe that his medication was not giving him any relief. He also had stomach pains, diarrhea and swelling in his face and hands. He was becoming extremely irritable and weak. His mother was a vegetarian and included many alternatives to animal proteins in Danny's diet. He ate plenty of nuts (almonds, cashews), seeds (sunflower, sesame) soybeans, and whole grains. When we tested him we found that he was deficient in minerals, especially magnesium and potassium, which were contained in all the foods that he was eating regularly, especially the nuts, seeds, soybeans, and whole grains. After the first seven basic treatments, he was treated for mineral mix. He had to be treated three times for mineral mix, then for magnesium. After he cleared for magnesium he no longer had any asthmatic symptoms or diarrhea. It wasn't until he was treated for potassium, however, that the swelling in his hands and face subsided, and his irritability and weakness disappeared. He can eat a vegetarian diet now without any reactions.

9. Salt Mix (sodium and sodium chloride, table salt, sea salt, rock salt, iodized salt, water softener salts, and chemicals).

You may use distilled water for drinking and washing, cooked rice, cooked grains, fresh or cooked vegetables and fruits (except celery, and onions; avoid canned or preserved vegetables and vegetable products) meats, chicken, and sugar.

Andrew, four-years-old, loved pretzels. His mother had been giving him pretzels since he began teething and continued to give them to him as a snack. He took a bag of pretzels with him to preschool and always had some in the car for long trips. The whole family loved them. Andrew was always running to the bathroom. His preschool teacher complained that he would have many accidents in class. He often wet the bed at night. His mother thought he would grow out of it. Then Andrew began to get irritable and complained of pain in his head. He wasn't behaving in class and was annoying his brothers and sister. After testing Andrew, we found that the salt on the pretzels he was eating was causing his symptoms. He was highly allergic to iodized salt and needed to be treated for salt alone and in combination with organs (his kidney meridian was blocked). Once he cleared his treatment he no longer wet his bed at night or had accidents at preschool. He became the kind, happy, helpful boy everyone knew. Actually the whole family was allergic to iodized salt! After treatment his mother was able to take her wedding ring off for the first time in years. She said she tried to take it off to clean it but her fingers had become so fat. Andrew's father's headaches cleared up as soon as he passed the salt treatment.

10. Corn Mix and Grain mix (blue corn, yellow corn, cornstarch, corn silk, corn syrup; wheat, gluten, corn, oats, millet, barley, kamut, couscous, farina, and brown rice). In some cases you may be able to treat corn and grains together at one time. Please check with your practitioner for the possibility of treating together. In severe allergies, they should be treated separately.

You may eat steamed or cooked vegetables, rice, fish, chicken, and meat. You may drink milk, water, tea and/or coffee. Avoid cream or sugar (corn may be a fortified ingredient in them).

Marty would return from school by 5:00 P.M. every evening. By 7:00 P.M. he will be covered with huge hives. By 10:00 P.M.. they would fade off. Marty's hives became a mystery to the family. Since hives hid not itch, hurt, or interfere with his daily activities, no one was concerned about them much. Then all of a sudden, he began feeling hot and itched whenever he had hives. He saw his family doctor and began taking antihistamine. Everyone thought the cause of the hives to be an allergy to mosquitos, since they came on in the evening and they had mosquitos around the house. He was referred to our office by his classmate's mother to be treated for insects. In our office, he was found to be allergic to most foods rather than insects. He bagan treatments for NAET basics. When he was treated for corn mix, within the first few minutes of the treatment, he got hives all over. He felt hot and restless. NAET for corn had to be repeated every five minutes for 11 times. By the end of 11 treatments, his hives diminished and he became normal. He was very allergic to corn. After this incidence, he shared with us that almost every evening when he returned from school, he would snack on corn chips and salsa. So it was the allergy to corn that caused his mysterious evening hives, not the mosquitos.

Grain Mix
You may eat vegetables, potato, fruits, meats, milk, and drink water. Avoid all products with gluten and grains.

Russell, fourteen, was very studious. He was a straight A student and had received many academic awards in school. But he always had stomach problems. He had colic as a baby and often would be constipated or have diarrhea. Russell began losing weight, was running a fever and had severe stomach pains after last Christmas. His mother thought he had the flu. After the family doctor examined Russell, he said that the symptoms could be due to colitis and more tests would be necessary. Russell continued to lose weight, had bouts of fever along with pains in the abdomen, painful, and irregular stools. He was given steroids and was hospitalized for three weeks, being fed intravenously. The doctors told Russell's mother he would have to stay on steroids indefinitely. His school work suffered. At the first sign of stress he would get sick. His whole life changed. He was placed on special diets, herbal medicines, vitamins, but nothing worked. When we first saw him he weighted 86 pounds. He was so weak his father carried him in to my office. Russell was severely allergic to all grains, especially rice, which he was being given to eat 6 times a day to stop the diarrhea. We began the treatments immediately. His symptoms began to subside after B complex. By the time he cleared the treatment for sugar his intense pain had disappeared and he gained a few pounds. It wasn't until he was treated for grains that the biggest change in his health occurred. He had to be treated separately for each grain. Several, especially rice, had to have multiple treatments and treatments with combinations. After clearing for all the grains, Russell gained weight, no longer had any fevers or stomach pains. His constant diarrhea was gone and he no longer needed to take steroids. He is a healthy straight-A student again!

11. Yeast Mix (brewer's yeast, torula yeast, bakers yeast, candia, yogurt, whey).
Whey
You may eat rice, vegetables, fruits, chicken, egg, turkey, beef, pork, beans, and lamb.
Yogurt
You may eat vegetables, meat, chicken, and fish. No fruits, no sugar products. Drink distilled water.

Six-year-old Marsha was always scratching her arms and legs. Her mother would put lotions and ointments on Marsha, but the rashes would not go away. She had deep cuts on the palms of her hands and whenever she put her hands in water or got them wet they would burn. The pediatrician prescribed a steroid cream to put on her skin twice a day. After Christmas Marsha's mother noticed that the rash was spreading. She mentioned it to her neighbor, a patient of ours, and she suggested that Marsha's mother make an appointment to see us. During the holidays Marsha visited her grandmother who loved to bake delicious breads, sweet rolls and cakes. Her breads had won first prize at the county fair. It was also Marsha's birthday and all her favorite treats were baked for her. We muscle tested and found that she was reacting to the baker's yeast in the breads and pastries she was eating. Her favorite food at home was pizza, which she had at least twice a week. She also had pizza once a week for lunch at school. The yeast in the pizza, breads and pastries were the cause of her red cracked, itchy skin rashes. After the ten basic treatments, she was treated for yeast mix and her skin rashes subsided.

Collect a small portion of different food groups from every meal and treat for the mixture of breakfast, lunch and dinner. Collect this combined food sample at least four times a month and treat using NAET.

12. Artificial Sweeteners (Sweet and Low, Equal, saccharine, Twin, and aspartame). There are many kinds of artificial sweeteners available today, which are refined and can affect and irritate the brain.

You may eat: anything without artificial sweeteners. Use freshly prepared items only.

Mario was five-years-old when his mother brought him to our office. He was very aggressive, angry, and had severe headaches. He fought with his brother and bit his younger sister's leg. His kindergarten teacher told his mother he wasn't ready for school and would not let him back in the classroom until his aggressive behavior stopped. His mother did not want to medicate him, as her pediatrician suggested, so she hoped we could help Mario. Muscle testing showed he was allergic to all the basic food groups. With each treatment his behavior improved, but his headaches were still severe. Whenever he had a headache he would become impossible to control. We asked his mother to write down the foods Mario was eating and found that his mother had eliminated sugar in her desserts and was substituting an artifi-

cial sweetener, trying to keep the refined sugar to a minimum. Mario was allergic to the artificial sweetener, which was giving him the headaches and causing his aggressive behavior. He needed repeated treatments before he cleared for artificial sweeteners. He is attending school now and his teacher is so pleased that he works and plays well with the other boys and girls in his class.

13. Coffee Mix (coffee, chocolate, caffeine, tannic acid, cocoa, cocoa butter, and carob). A caffeine- like substance is secreted by certain parts of the brain, and is very essential for its normal function. If the child is allergic to any of these, it can irritate the brain.

You may consume anything that has no coffee, caffeine, chocolate and/or carob.

Mark, ten-years-old, developed a rash all over his body: on his face, the sides of his cheeks, the palms of his hands, behind his neck and ears. His mother took him to a dermatologist, who prescribed topical creams and gave Mark a mild lotion to wash with instead of the soap he was using. The creams gave him some temporary relief, but the rash continued to itch. It kept him up through the night. He was tired during the day and couldn't concentrate on his school work. His mother made an appointment to see me after reading a magazine article about NAET. Mark was allergic to the basic ten food groups as well as caffeine. Mark said he never drank coffee or tea. He only drank caffeine-free soda. After muscle testing, I told Mark that his rash was coming from something he was having everyday that had caffeine in it. Mark and his mother went through the foods he ate each day. After school he would have milk and chocolate chip cookies or Oreo before he started his homework. After dinner while watching television, he had frozen yogurt- chocolate or coffee flavored. I told Mark to substitute different flavored cookies and frozen yogurt until he could be treated for caffeine and we began the basic treatments. When they returned the next week his face was not as red and his neck was clear. When he completed all the basic treatments and the treatment for Caffeine Mix, his skin became normal again; he slept through the night; and his schoolwork improved.

14. Spice Mix 1: (ginger, cardamon, cinnamon cloves, nutmeg, garlic, cumin, fennel, coriander, turmeric, saffron, and mint). You may use all foods and products without these items.

12-year-old Joe suffered from repeated ear infection and pain inside the ear for almost two years on and off. He had various treatments for that. But his problem continued. When we examined him we found that his earache and infection were due to a particular spice he was eating every day. Probing into his daily diet, it was found that his favorite cereal was "Cinnamon crunch," and he ate that every morning. He was free of earaches and repeated infection after he was treated for that spice successfully.

Spice Mix 2 (peppers, red pepper, black pepper, green pepper, jalapeno, banana peppers, anise seed, basil, bay leaf, caraway seed, chervil, cream of tartar, dill, fenugreek, horseradish, mace, MSG, mustard, onion, oregano, paprika, ginger, poppy seed, parsley, rosemary, sage, sumac, and vinegar).
You may eat or use all foods and food products without the above listed spices.

Mindy's family drank ginger tea every day after supper because they thought it was good for digestion. Seven year old Mindy tried ginger tea with honey one day and she too liked the taste of it. Ever since she began drinking ginger tea every night. Within a week, she developed severe pains in the joints. Worried parents took her to the doctor. The doctor didn't have any explanation for this sudden arthritic pain. He sent her home with some anal-gesics and antiinflammatory drugs. She continued to drink gin-ger tea every day. Her pain kept getting worse day by day and she couldn't go to school for a number of days. According to her teacher's suggestion, she was brought to our office. She was car-ried in to the office because she couldn't walk due to pain. By testing with NTT, ginger tea was found to be the culprit for her debilitating pain. She was treated immediately for ginger and within 30 minutes her joints loosened up and she was free of pain. She walked home. Later she was treated for all the basic 25 groups. She is a healthy, happy girl now.

15. Animal Fat (butter, lard, chicken fat, beef fat, lamb fat, and fiish oil).

You may use anything other than the above including veg-etable oils.

Twelve-year-old Josh suffered from severe painful acne and dry skin. He was involved in so many after school activities that he hardly had any time to eat with his family. He was always stopping for a quick bite at a fast food restaurant for a ham-burger and fries or some fried chicken. When he was tested we found that he was allergic to the animal fats and fatty acids in his diet. His skin began clearing up as soon as he completed his treatment for fats. It is no longer dry and Josh can enjoy his hamburger and fries without a reaction.

Vegetable Fat (corn oil, canola oil, peanut oil, linseed oil, sunflower oil, palm oil, flax seed oil, and coconut oil).

You may use steamed vegetables, steamed rice, meats, eggs, chicken, butter, and animal fats.

16. Nut Mix 1 (peanuts, black walnuts, or English walnuts). You may eat any foods that do not contain the nuts listed above including their oils and butter.

Nut Mix 2 (cashew, almonds, pecan, Brazil nut, hazelnut, macadamia nut, and sunflower seeds). You may eat any foods that do not contain the nuts listed above including their oils and butters.

17. Fish Mix (Cod, halibut, salmon, shark, and tuna). You may eat any food that does not contain the fish or fish oils listed above.

Shellfish Mix (Shrimp, lobster, abalone, cray, crab, and clams). You may eat any food that does not contain fish products.

My Allergy to Shellfish

I just wanted to let you know that 7 years ago I became allergic to seafood, including shellfish and fish after having a sea kelp wrap at a Spa in Florida. I grew up in Bar Harbor, Maine and ate seafood all my life! Recently I went to Dr. Alexander, Alexander Chiropractic Center in Lawrenceville, GA and was treated (it took 4 times), but I can now eat shrimp, clams, scallops, etc. and I no longer break out in hives all over my body! The hives I used to get were big welts and lasted sometimes up to 2-3 weeks before they finally cleared up. What a blessing this is. I was also allergic to Vitamin C and Chocolate and stomach acid. Life has certainly improved! Thank you for finding this technology.

Sincerly,
Martha Fleck
Suwanee, GA

18. Amino Acids-1 (essential amino acids: lysine, methionine, leucine, threonine, valine, tryptophane, isoleucine, and phenylalanine).
You may eat cooked white rice, lettuce, and boiled chicken.

Amino Acids 2 (non essential amino acids: alanine, arginine, aspartic acid, carnitine citrulline, cysteine, glutamic acid, glycine, histidine, ornithine, proline, serine, taurine, and tyrosine).
You may eat cooked white rice, cauliflower, boiled beef (corned beef), and iceberg lettuce.

19. Whiten All
You may eat cooked vegetables, pasta, rice, meats, chicken, and eggs.

20. Turkey (Serotonin)
You may eat any food that does not contain B1, B3, B6, tryptophane, and neurotransmitters (dopamine, epinephrine, norepinephrine, serotonin, acetylcholine).

Susan, eleven-years-old, was having difficulty sleeping through the night. She would get up three to four times a night and couldn't get back to sleep. She was withdrawn, didn't want to participate in any activities and was depressed. The school counselor started seeing her on a regular basis, but she couldn't snap out of her depression and sleeplessness. She had many food and environmental allergies so we began the basic ten treatments. It wasn't until we muscle tested for turkey that we discovered she was allergic to serotonin. An allergy to serotonin can cause sleep disturbances and depression. Since turkey is a healthy meat, her mother fed her turkey sandwich everyday. We had to treat Susana three times before she passed the treatment for turkey and serotonin. She no longer sees the school counselor. She sleeps through the night and has joined the after-school drama class.

21. Fluoride

You may use or eat: fruits, poultry, meat, potato, cauliflower, white rice, and yellow vegetables. You may use distilled water, drink fresh fruit juices.

22. Gum Mix (Acacia, Karaya gum, Xanthine gum, black gum, sweet gum, and chewing gum).

You may eat rice, pasta, vegetables, fruits without skins, meats, eggs, and chicken, drink juice and water.

23. Dried bean Mix (vegetable proteins, soybean, and lecithin).

You may eat rice, pasta, vegetables, meats, eggs, and anything other than beans and bean products.

Sharon a fourteen-year-old gymnast was suffering from a painful low backache. She couldn't practice for the up coming exhibition. The pain was so intense her physician had given her instructions to stay in bed and take muscle relaxers. Through muscle testing we found that it was something she was eating for three or four days. Her aunt was visiting and had made a huge pot of lentil soup, which was Sharon's favorite. She had been eating some at lunch and dinner for several days. She was treated for the lentil soup and the next day, after the twenty-five hour waiting period was over her backache was gone.

24. Alcohol (candy, ice cream, liquid medication in alcohol, and alcohol).

You may eat vegetables, meats, fish eggs, and chicken.

25. Gelatin

You may use anything that does not contain gelatin.

26. Vegetable mix

27. Vitamin D.
You may eat fruits, vegetables, poultry, and meats.

28. Vitamin E.
You may eat fresh fish, carrots, potato, poultry, and meat.

29. Vitamin F (vegetable oils, wheat germs oils, linseed oil, sunflower oil, soybean oil, safflower oil, flax seed oil, clarified butter, grape seed oil, and peanut oil.
You may eat anything that does not contain any of the above oils.

30. Vitamin T
You may eat fish, rice, potato, poultry, and meat.

31. RNA & DNA (Please refer to the guidebook for details).

32. Stomach acid (Hydrochloric acid).
You may eat raw and steamed vegetables, cooked dried beans, eggs, oils, clarified butter, and milk.

Martha, thirteen-years-old, suffered from acid reflux. She was extremely thin and couldn't hold any food down after eating. During her NTT evaluation, she told me that ten minutes after eating anything, she felt highly acidic and had to throw up. She was allergic to her own stomach acid. She was treated for stomach acid immediately and sent home. When she returned the following week, she had a big smile on her face. Her acid reflux had stopped the day after her treatment for stomach acid.

33. Base (digestive juice from the intestinal tract contains various digestive enzymes: amylase, protease, lipase, maltase, peptidase, bromelain, cellulase, sucrase, papain, lactase, gluco-amylase, and alpha galactosidase).

You may eat acid producing foods: sugars, starches, grains, breads, and meats.

Sam, ten-years-old, complained of severe abdominal bloating for two-three hours after eating. He was very uncomfortable and became very irritable and angry with his friends and family. He couldn't fall asleep at night, staying up until two o'clock in the morning. He had to get up by five-thirty to get ready for school. He was always tired and began hating to eat. He was allergic to his digestive juices. When he was successfully treated for Base (intestinal digestive juices), his abdominal bloating, insomnia, and irritability stopped.

34. Food colors (different food colors in many sources like: ice cream, candy, cookie, gums, drinks, spices, other foods, and/or lipsticks, etc.).

You may eat foods that are freshly prepared. Avoid carrots, natural spices, beets, berries, frozen green leafy vegetables like spinach.

Ten-year-old Cindy suffered from severe sinusitis, ever since she started going to school. She was taking allergy shots for two years but her sinuses were always getting infected. She was very artistic and since kindergarten loved to draw. She craved jelly beans and puddings and ice-creams. Through muscle testing we found out that the food colorings in the crayons, jelly beans and ice creams were giving her sinusitis. After treating her for food colorings her sinuses cleared and she no longer receives allergy shots.

35. Food additives (sulfates, nitrates, BHT).

You cannot eat hotdog or any prepackaged food. Eat anything made at home from scratch.

Every Monday morning, six-year-old Ryan would have a sore throat and an earache. At first his mother thought that he didn't want to go to school after being home for the weekend. He began running a fever, so his mother took him to the family doctor. The doctor examined Ryan's ears and told his mother that it might be necessary to put tubes in his ears. His mother came to see us before agreeing to put the tubes in Ryan's ears. Since his earaches happened every Monday morning we asked what type of activities and foods Ryan participated in on the weekends. Every Sunday the family would go to the park. There was a petting zoo there with a hot dog stand next to it. Ryan would have a hotdog every Sunday evening. He was allergic to the food additives in the hot dog. His earaches disappeared when he cleared his treatment to food additives.

36. Refined starches (corn starch, potato starch, and modified starch). Refined starches are used as a thickening agent in sauces and drinks. Many people are allergic to starches. Refined starches should be avoided.

You may eat whole grains, vegetables, meats, chicken, and fish.

Baking powder/ Baking soda (in baked goods, toothpaste, and/or detergents).

You may eat or use anything that does not contain baking powder or baking soda including fresh fruits, vegetables, fats, meat, and chicken.

37. Night shade vegetables: Tomato, potato, eggplant, bell pepper and onion make up the nightshade vegetable group. Most people are missing the enzyme in their bodies that helps with the digestion of this special chemical contained in these vegetables. After treatment, the body will begin to produce the special enzyme to digest these vegetables.

Avoid eating these vegetables while you treat.

38. Virus mix

Avoid contact with people with any infection. Avoid uncooked foods, old and stale food. Eat freshly cooked food and drink freshly boiled cooled water. Distilled water is not sufficient to replace freshly boiled cooled water.

39. Bacteria Mix

Avoid contact with people with any infection. Avoid uncooked foods, old and stale food. Eat freshly cooked food and drink freshly boiled cooled water. Distilled water is not always safe. People have developed sickness from distilled water bought in sealed bottles from the store.

Ten-year-old Natasha suffered from severe painful boils all over her body since the age of two. She was given various antibiotics several times, cortisone creams to apply locally but none of these had lasting results. Her boils kept under control as long as she took the antibiotics. They returned right back the day after she stopped the antibiotics. The old boils grew as large as a red grape and burst at the top releasing yellow pus healing by next day or so. The healing one looked like a cross sectioned red onion for a few days, peeling and sloughing, eventually forming a scab. Then the scab fell off leaving a scar. The new ones continued to erupt almost every day at any surface of the body. Sometimes on her face, sometimes on her chest, back, inner thighs, around vagina, vulva, rectum, etc. She was not only in physical pain also in emotional pain and embarrassment to be with her classmates. Finally, her mother began home-school with her. When we examined her, she was found to be allergic to all the NAET basics. She began treatments right away for the basics. After the vitamin C, her boils were reduced in size and less painful. The new eruptions were not so much angry looking. After basic ten she was treated for bacteria mix and a combination of bacteria mix and vitamin C. A week after the treatment for bacteria and vitamin C, she reported that all boils healed suddenly. After two years, she still hasn't seen the return of her boils. Most of her scars also healed nicely without leaving marks on the skin or disfiguring her. She is a beautiful, healthy, teenager now.

40. Parasites

Many people host various parasites in the body. They find their way into our body via uncooked vegetables, meats, fish and unwashed fruits. Once when they get in they multiply rapidly and find their way into the blood stream. Parasite infestation can cause various health disorders in the body, including upper respiratory infections, asthma, brain fatigue, brain fog, fibromyalgia, insomnia, general itching, abdominal bloating, pain in the abdomen, sinusitis, diarrhea, anal itching, hyperactivity, irritability, mood swings, and unexplained weight gain.

Marian was eight and chubby looking. She was fifteen pounds over weight. Her mother said she was very skinny before her last vacation to Cabo San Lucas. After she returned, she complained of nausea every so often, poor appetite, extreme thirst, and weight gain. She was tested for hypothyroidism, diabetes, and various other tests. No abnormalities were traced except overweight. She was put on a low calorie diet. In our office she was found to be allergic to a few basic food groups. She was also found to be allergic to parasites. Her stool was sent out to the lab. She had pinworms.

She was treated for all NAET basics and parasites. She was placed on some herbs. Her health improved, her appetite improved and above all she lost her excess weight.

Water (drinking water, tap water, filtered water, city water, lake water, rain water, ocean water, and river water).

People can react to any water. Treat them as needed and avoid the item treated.

Sharon had developed a severe case of eczema six months before her mother brought her to us for evaluation and treatment. She always was becoming hyperactive and had difficulty sitting still in school or focusing on her schoolwork. After testing her by NTT, we found that she had an allergy to the water she was drinking. Her mother had installed a new water filtration system in their house six months before. The water softener was the culprit causing her eczema and irritability. Her skin and personality became normal when she cleared for the water.

41. Chemicals (chlorine, swimming pool water, detergents, fabric softeners, soaps, cleaning products, shampoos, lipsticks, and cosmetics you or other family members use).

Avoid the above items.

Tom, was the best player on his water polo team in high school. He always scored the crucial points at the end of the game. His mother, one of our patients, told me that he always felt dizzy after a game. He was complaining of joint pains and for the last year would have migraine headaches, which lasted for days. He was missing more and more days of school. I asked his mother to keep track of his symptoms and she made an appointment to bring him in the following week. When I examined Tom, his ears were clogged and his sinuses were congested. Tom had kept a record of his symptoms for the week: Tuesday, Thursday, and Saturday mornings he woke up with a headache and joint pains. He said that the mornings are the most difficult for him. His sinuses and ears always hurt. Monday, Wednesday, and Friday he had dizzy spells. Tom's water polo team practiced every Monday, Wednesday and Friday in the school pool. The chemicals in the swimming pool water were giving Tom all the headaches, joint pains, dizzy spells, ear and sinus infections. He was highly allergic to the chlorine in the water. Chlorine may be a disinfectant keeping most of the bacteria and viruses out of the water, but it can do serious harm to anyone sensitive to it. We treated Tom for chlorine immediately and asked him to bring a sample of his school's pool water with him on his next visit. It took six treatments for Tom to clear for his school's pool water. Finally, after he had passed, his headaches, joint pains, and ear and sinuses congestion disappeared.

Inhalants
Avoid pollens, weeds, grasses, flowers, wood mix, room air, outside air, smog, and polluted air from nearby factories.

Nicola, nine-years-old used an inhaler two or three times a day because her asthma was so severe. Once or twice a month she had to be taken to the emergency room and placed on the hospital's inhaler. She had no energy, had lost weight and was always catching a cold or flu. Her symptoms started two years back when her family moved to the beach. Through NTT, I discovered that she was reacting to mold and fungus around her home. After treating her for mold mix, she only used her inhaler once or twice a week. She collected mold and fungus from her house and adjacent yard and brought it to the clinic. After passing the treatment for the mold and fungus in her home, she no longer needed an inhaler at all. She gained weight and now runs and plays with her friends.

Allergic to Grasses, Weeds, and Pollens
Francine, 6-years-old was spending the summer with her grandmother, who lived on a farm in the mid-west. She had never been out of the city before and was very excited. Her parents were going to be traveling and were happy that Francine would have so many exciting things to do in the farm. From the moment she arrived, she loved the green hills and all

the animals. She would get up at dawn and help with feeding the chickens and even tried milking the cows. The peaches were ready for picking and she would climb up the ladder a pick the ripest ones. A few weeks after Francine arrived she woke up congested. The next day she was coughing and sneezing. Her grandmother kept her inside for a few days and her coughing quieted down. It was time to pick the corn and Francine didn't want to miss out. As soon as she began to pick out the the corn her cough returned. By that evening her throat was sore. Her grandmother was very worried and took her to the doctor who gave her some cough medicine and told her to rest. Her parents were coming to take her home in a few days and her grandmother wanted her to be well by then. However, when her parents saw her she was much worse, wheezing, tired and running a fever. Francine's cold turned into bronchitis and it was getting more and more severe. When her mother brought her to the office she had lost weight, had dark circles under eyes and was very pale. We found Francine to be allergic to weeds, pollens, grasses, animal dander, feathers, corn, trees, molds and fungus along with the basic 10 food groups. Her mother said that they never considered that Francine had allergies because she didn't exhibit any symptoms at home. Going to the country overloaded Francine's immune system with allergens that her body couldn't fight off. She was treated for all the basic foods, pollens, trees, grasses, molds and fungus. She was off again to visit her grandmother next summer. She telephoned me as soon as she returned from her trip to say she hadn't had one allergic reaction, not a cough or a sniffle.

43. Grasses and Weeds

44. Formaldehyde

Fabrics (daily and sleep attire; towels, bed linens, blankets, formaldehyde).

Treat each kind of fabric separately and avoid the particular cloth or kind of cloth for 25 hours.

When Denise bought her new born baby into the clinic she was hysterical. After seeing her pediatrician, she didn't know what to do. Katlin, her three-week-old baby had an oozing rash on her body and cried and screamed throughout the night, whether she was fed or not. Her doctor told her that he really couldn't find anything wrong with the baby, and gave her some medication and an ointment for the rash. The baby continued to scream through the night. Using the mother as a surrogate we muscle tested and found Katlin to be allergic to cotton, which was in just about everything the baby touched. Her mother said she only used cotton sheets and blankets, even cotton diapers because she wanted the purest fabrics near the baby. We treated the baby through the mother. The next morning Denise called the clinic and said she and her baby had their first night's sleep since they came home from the hospital. She brought the baby back the following week to show me how lovely her skin was. She was wearing a pretty pink cotton baby kimono and cooing happily.

45. Latex products (shoe, sole of the shoe, elastic, rubber bands, and/or rubber bathtub toys, computer parts, certain household items, certain cosmetic products, elastics on various products, clothes, work materials, etc.).
Avoid latex products.

Three year-old Diana's face was covered with eczema. Eczema was spreading through the face including: around the mouth, both cheeks, forehead, nose, eyelids. She was on various medications, one for itching, one for pain, one to prevent infection, etc. In spite of all medications and care she received, for the past 2 years and 8 months she suffered from this disorder.

In our office NTT testing revealed that she was simply allergic to latex. Her pacifier and nipples of her feeding bottles were the source. She cleared her eczema completely after she was treated for latex.

Plastics (toys, play or work materials, utensils, toiletries, computer key boards, and/or phone).
Avoid contact with products made from plastics. Wear a pair of cotton gloves.

46. Crude oil/Synthetic materials
School work materials (crayons, coloring paper and books, inks, pencils, crayons, glue, play dough, other arts, and craft materials).
Avoid using them or contacting them. Wear a pair of gloves if you have to go near them.

Four-year-old, Matt refused to obey his parents. He threw his crayons and coloring books around, tore out pages and ran around the house. His mother tried everything to calm him, but he wouldn't sit still for a minute. She brought him to the clinic. We tested him and found that he was allergic to food colorings, crayons and coloring books and picture books that had colored illustrations. He loved red candies and jelly beans. He became much calmer after he cleared for food coloring. Once he cleared for crayons and books he was able to sit quietly and color without any interruption or negative behaviors.

48. Smoking/Nicotine

49. Dust/dustmites

50. Flower mix.

Drugs given in infancy, during childhood or taken by the mother during pregnancy (antibiotics, sedatives, laxatives, or recreational drugs).
Avoid the drug.

Amy, seven-years-old, was living with her grandmother who brought her to our clinic from the east coast. She was having trouble learning to read in school. Her teacher was recommending that she be placed in a special education class. Her grandmother told us that her parents took recreational drugs before Amy was born. I tested Amy and found that even though she had never had any recreational drugs, she was highly allergic to them. Her mother had passed them on to her during her pregnancy. She also was allergic to the basic food groups, food additives and preservatives. We treated Amy every day during her three week stay. She became ill during the treatment for drugs, running a fever and having chills. When she cleared the drug treatment she was much calmer. We received a letter from her grandmother after they returned home saying that Amy's teacher couldn't believe the difference in her. She was alert, attentive, and focused. Amy was sounding out words and reading aloud. They couldn't be happier. They are planning to return during the school break to complete the treatments.

Immunizations and vaccinations either you received or your parent received before you were born (DPT, POLIO, MMR, small pox, chicken pox, influenza, or hepatitis).
Nothing to avoid except infected persons or recently inoculated persons if there are any near you.

Allergy to DPT Immunization
Jimmy was a bright happy toddler until he was about 18 months old his mother told me as she was trying to keep him from throwing his toys all over my office. He was unable to sit still, would rock back and forth, and would not respond to any

questions. At 3 years of age he was unable to say his name. His mother told me he was speaking and counting to ten when he was a year old. She didn't know what to do now that the pediatrician and specialist diagnosed him as having autism. Jimmy was allergic to all the basic food groups and environmental allergens. With each treatment his behavior improved, but he was not responding to any questions we asked. Investigating further I asked his mother if she remembered anything unusual that might have happened to him as a toddler. She said he didn't really have any severe childhood illness, but he did have a high fever that lasted a few weeks after his DPT immunization. We tested through his mother and found that Jimmy was severely allergic to the DPT shot and immediately treated him. He had an immediate reaction to the treatment and became uncontrollable. I quickly retreated him again and had to do so every ten minutes for one hour before he calmed down. Jimmy was so sensitive to the DPT that it was necessary to treat each component separately, (diphtheria, tetanus and pertussis). After clearing each component Jimmy began responding to our questions with yes and no answers. He now is in kindergarten and is a normal well adjusted 5-year-old.

The items listed below are treated as needed and on a priority based protocol, which your NAET practitioner will explain to you.

Histamine

Whenever there is an allergic reaction in the body, special cells (mast cells) release histamine. You can be allergic to your own histamine. When that happens, histamine is produced very frequently in the body. It doesn't stop until the mechanism is turned off. Another way to turn to turn off histamine is to take antihistamine, either in a medication or a natural way with vitamin C (that is if you are not allergic to it). It is very easy to treat for your own histamine with NAET, then your body will adjust to your histamine by itself to a normal level.

Gina was allergic to all the major food groups and environmental allergens. Her mother had taken the nine-year-old to every specialist in her area because Gina's reactions were so intense she would have to rush her to the emergency room for intravenous adrenaline and steroids to stop her swelling. Her throat, mouth, face, hands, feet would fill up with liquids moments after she came in contact with an allergen. After exercising at school, Gina's face swelled so much that you couldn't see her nose. The school called the paramedics at once. Her mother brought Gina to us after reading, Say Good-bye to Illness. Yes, Gina was allergic to her own histamine, as well as foods and environmental allergens. We immediately treated her for histamine. She needed ten treatments, ten minutes apart before she held the treatment. Her swelling was reduced with each treatment. After clearing for histamine her allergic reactions became much less severe and were no longer life threatening. She has been receiving treatments for a year and a half now and is no longer on any medication and can eat from the basic food groups without any difficulties. She exercises in school without any reactions at all.

Heavy metals (mercury, lead, cadmium, aluminum, arsenic, copper, gold, silver, and vanadium).

You may use only distilled water for drinking, washing and showering. You may eat only cooked rice, vegetables, fruits, meats, eggs, milk, coffee, and tea.

Martha, fourteen, had severe neck and shoulder pains. She was on the school volleyball team and was always taking aspirin to relieve the pain. Her mother was a patient at our clinic and brought Martha to see us. Through muscle testing we discovered that she was allergic to the gold chain she had received as a birthday present. She loved the locket her parents gave her so much that she never took it off. She said it was her good luck charm and she played much better with it. We immediately treated her for the gold chain and locket. The next day they returned after the twenty-five hour waiting period. Martha was smiling, saying she didn't need to take any aspirin to relief her pain. She had passed the treatment for the chain and locket. She wears her good luck necklace everyday now, without any neck or shoulder pain.

Hormones (estrogen, progesterone, testosterone).
You may eat vegetables, fruits, grains, chicken, and fish.

Neurotransmitters (dopamine, epinephrine, norepinephrine, serotonin, acetylcholine).
You may eat anything other than milk products, and turkey.

MSG (monosodium glutamate).
You may eat freshly prepared vegetables, fruits, meat, and grains without MSG.

Paper Products (newspaper, ink, reading books, coloring books, with colored illustrations)
Avoid the above items.

Perfume (room deodorizers, soaps, flowers, perfumes, or after-shave, etc.).
Avoid perfume and any fragrance from flowers or products containing perfume.

Julie and her husband, Doug brought their four-month-old baby to the clinic with a curious complaint. Every time Doug was near the baby up, he would cry. It didn't matter if he was feeding him, playing with him or just holding him. Doug picked the baby and sure enough he started crying. Through muscle testing we checked everything Doug was wearing, but the baby wasn't allergic to anything her father was wearing. He wasn't allergic to his father; he was allergic to his after-shave lotion. We treated the baby through his mother. Mother, father and baby are enjoying one another now.

Pesticides (malathion, termite control items, or regular pesticides).

Avoid meats, grasses, ant sprays, and pesticides.

Twelve-year-old Jenny, was brought to our office with a curious complaint, she would get congested, cough and wheeze, only when she was in her bedroom. Using NTT, her symptoms were tied to a chemical that was used in her room. Jenny's room was in the original part of the house, which was forty-five years old. Her mother remembered that they had that part of the house sprayed for termites. Jenny was treated for pesticides and after clearing could stay in her room without getting congested, coughing or wheezing.

Insect bites in infancy or childhood (bee, ant, wasp, spider, or cockroach, etc.).

Treat for the individual insect and avoid it while treating.

Austin, eight-years-old came home from school complaining that his arm hurt. His mother didn't notice anything wrong at first, but by Austin's bedtime his arm had become red and swollen. She washed it and put some disinfectant on it, but couldn't find a cut or bruise. In the middle of the night Austin woke up with a fever. His mother gave him Tylenol. She took him to the doctor in the morning who prescribed an antibiotic and said it looked as though Austin was bitten by a spider or wasp. Five days of taking antibiotics didn't bring the swelling down at all. By the time we saw Austin he was very ill. He was allergic to the spider bite. We treated him immediately. The swelling was reduced within minutes after the treatment.

Radiation (computer, television, microwave, X-ray, and the sun).
Avoid radiation of any kind.

Dominic, ten-years-old, had a history of canker sores whenever he walked in the sun. He turned out to be allergic to vitamin D, (one of the vitamins produced in the body with the help of sunlight). After he was treated by NAET for vitamin D, the incidence of canker sores after being exposed to the sun diminished.

Tissues and secretions (DNA, RNA, thyroid hormone, pituitary hormone, pineal gland, hypothalamus, or brain tissue, liver, blood, and saliva).

Allergies to people, animals and pets (mother, father, care takers, cats, and dogs).
Avoid the ones you were treated for 25 hours.

Emotional allergies (fear, fright, frustration, anger, low self-esteem, and/or rejection, etc.).
Nothing to avoid for emotional treatment.

After clearing the allergy to nutrients, appropriate supplementation with vitamins, minerals, and enzymes etc., is necessary to make up the deficiency and promote healing. Please read the guidebook for information on how to take supplement correctly. Your NAET doctor will also do a few energy boosting techniques with vitamin B complex, calcium, vitamin F, neurotransmitters, sugar, trace minerals, and magnesium. Ask your NAET practitioner about boosting techniques.

It will be a good idea to have your young ones to get treated (if there is an allergy) for nicotine, tobacco, different liquors, alcohol, illicit drugs, etc., so that when they grow up if they happened to get exposed to these products they may not have any craving towards it. If they don't have an allergy, they may not get tempted to use them and they may remain healthy and productive people forever.

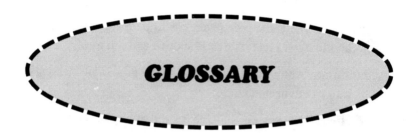

GLOSSARY

GLOSSARY

Acetylcholine: A neurotransmitter manufactured in the brain, used for memory and control of sensory input and muscular output signals.

Acid: Any compound capable of releasing a hydrogen ion; it will have a pH of less than 7.

Acute: Extremely sharp or severe, as in pain can also refer to an illness or reaction that is sudden and intense.

Adaptation: Ability of an organism to integrate new elements into its environment.

Addiction: A dependent state characterized by cravings for a particular substance if that substance is withdrawn.

Additive: A substance added in small amounts to foods to alter the food in some way.

Adrenaline: Trademark for preparations of epinephrine, which is a hormone secreted by the adrenal gland. It is used sublingually and by injection to stop allergic reactions.

Aldehyde: A class of organic compounds obtained by oxidation of alcohol. Formaldehyde and acetaldehyde are members of this class of compounds.

Alkaline: Basic, or any substance that accepts a hydrogen ion; its pH will be greater than 7.

Allergenic: Causing or producing an allergic reaction.

Allergen: Any organic or inorganic substance from one's surroundings or from within the body itself that causes an allergic response in an individual is called an allergen. An allergen can cause an IgE antibody mediated or non-IgE mediated response in a person. Some of the commonly known allergens are: pollens, molds, animal dander, food and drinks, chemicals of different kind like the ones found in the food, water, air, fabrics, cleaning agents, environmental materials, detergent, make-up products etc., body secretions, bacteria, virus, synthetic materials, fumes, and air pollution. Emotional unpleasant thoughts like anger, frustration, etc can also become allergens and cause allergic reactions in people.

Allergic reaction: Adverse, varied symptoms, unique to each person, resulting from the body's response to exposure to allergens.

Allergy: Attacks by the immune system on harmless or even useful things entering the body. Abnormal responses to substances usually well tolerated by most people.

Amino acid: An organic acid that contains an amino (ammonia-like NH3) chemical group; the building blocks that make up all proteins.

Anaphylactic shock: Also known as anaphylaxis. Usually it happens suddenly when exposed to a highly allergic item. But sometimes, it can also happen as a cumulative reaction. (first two doses of penicillin may not trigger a severe reaction, but third or fourth one could produce an anaphylaxis in some people). An anaphylaxis (this life threatening allergic reaction) is characterized by: an immediate allergic reaction that can cause difficulty in breathing, light headedness, fainting, sensation of chills, internal cold, severe heart palpitation or irregular heart beats, pallor, eyes rolling, poor mental clarity, tremors, internal shaking, extreme fear, angio neurotic edema, throat swelling, drop in blood pressure, nausea, vomiting, diarrhea, swelling anywhere in the body, redness and hives, fever, delirium, unresponsiveness, or sometimes even death.

Antibody: A protein molecule produced in the body by lymphocytes in response to a perceived harmful foreign or abnormal substance (another protein) as a defense mechanism to protect the body.

Antigen: Any substance recognized by the immune system that causes the body to produce antibodies; also refers to a concentrated solution of an allergen.

Antihistamine: A chemical that blocks the reaction of histamine that is released by the mast cells and basophils during an allergic reaction. Any substance that slows oxidation, prevents damage from free radicals and results in oxygen sparing.

Assimilate: To incorporate into a system of the body; to transform nutrients into living tissue.

Autoimmune: A condition resulting when the body makes antibodies against its own tissues or fluid. The immune system attacks the body it inhabits, which causes damage or alteration of cell function.

Binder: A substance added to tablets to help hold them together.

Blood brain barrier: A cellular barrier that prevents certain chemicals from passing from the blood to the brain.

Candida albicans: A genus of yeast like fungi normally found in the body. It can multiply and cause infections, or toxicity.

Candidiasis: An overgrowth of Candida organisms, which are part of the normal flora of the mouth, skin, intestines and vagina.

Carbohydrate, complex: A large molecule consisting of simple sugars linked together, found in whole grains, vegetables, and fruits. This metabolizes slowly into glucose than refined carbohydrate.

Carbohydrate, refined: A molecule of sugar that metabolizes quickly to glucose. Refined white sugar, white rice, white flour are some of the examples.

Cerebral allergy: Mental dysfunction caused by sensitivity to foods, chemicals, environmental substances, or other substances like work materials etc.

Chronic: Of long duration.

Chronic fatigue syndrome: A syndrome of multiple symptoms most commonly associated with fatigue and reduced energy or no energy.

Crohn's disease: An intestinal disorder associated with irritable bowel syndrome, inflammation of the bowels and colitis.

Cumulative reaction: A type of reaction caused by an accumulation of allergens in the body.

Cytokine: A chemical produced by the T-cells during an infection as our immune system's second line of defense. Examples of cytokines are interleukin 2 and gamma interferon.

Desensitization: The process of building up body tolerance to allergens by the use of extracts of the allergenic substance.

Detoxification: A variety of methods used to reduce toxic materials accumulated in body tissues.

Digestive tract: Includes the salivary glands, mouth, esophagus, stomach, small intestine, portions of the liver, pancreas, and large intestine.

Disorder: A disturbance of regular or normal functions.

Dust: Dust Particles from various sources irritate sensitive individual causing different respiratory problems like asthma, bronchitis, hay-fever like symptoms, sinusitis, and cough.

Dust mites: Microscopic insects that live in dusty areas, pillows, blankets, bedding, carpets, upholstered furniture, drapes, corners of the houses where people neglect to clean regularly.

Eczema: An inflammatory process of the skin resulting from skin allergies causing dry, itchy, crusty, scaly, weepy, blisters or eruptions on the skin. skin rash frequently caused by allergy.

Edema: Excess fluid accumulation in tissue spaces. It could be localized or generalized.

Electromagnetic: Refers to emissions and interactions of both electric and magnetic components. Magnetism arising from electric charge in motion. This has a definite amount of energy.

Elimination diet: A diet in which common allergenic foods and those suspected of causing allergic symptoms have been temporarily eliminated.

Endocrine: refers to ductless glands that manufacture and secrete hormones into the blood stream or extracellular fluids.

Endogenous: Originating from or due to internal causes.

Environment: A total of circumstances and/or surroundings in which an organism exists. May be a combination of internal or external influences that can affect an individual.

Environmental illness: A complex set of symptoms caused by adverse reactions of the body to external and internal environments.

Enzyme: A substance, usually protein in nature and formed in living cells, which starts or stops biochemical reactions.

Eosinophil: A type of white blood cell. Eosinophil levels may be high in some cases of allergy or parasitic infestation.

Erythrocyte: Red blood cell.

Exocrine: Refers to substance released through ducts that lead to a body compartment or surface.

Exogenous: Originating from or due to external causes.

Extracellular: Situated outside a cell or cells.

Extract: Treatment dilution of an antigen used in immunotherapy, such as food, chemical, or pollen extract.

Fibromyalgia: An immune complex disorder causing general body aches, muscle aches, and general fatigue.

"Fight" or "flight": The activation of the sympathetic branch of the autonomic nervous system, preparing the body to meet a threat or challenge.

Food addiction: A person becomes dependent on a particular allergenic food and must keep eating it regularly in order to prevent withdrawal symptoms.

Food grouping: A grouping of foods according to their botanical or biological characteristics.

Gastrointestinal: Relating both to stomach and intestines.

Histamine: A body substance released by mast cells and basophils during allergic reactions, which precipitates allergic symptoms.

Holistic: Refers to the idea that health and wellness depend on a balance between physical (Structural) aspects, physiological (chemical, nutritional, functional) aspects, emotional and spiritual aspects of a person.

Homeopathic: Refers to giving minute amounts of remedies that in massive doses would produce effects similar to the condition being treated.

Homeostasis: A state of perfect balance in the organism also called as Yin-yang balance. The balance of functions and chemical composition within an organism that results from the actions of regulatory systems.

Hormone: A chemical substance that is produced in the body, secreted into body fluids, and is transported to other organs, where it produces a specific effect on metabolism.

Hypersensitivity: An acquired reactivity to an antigen that can result in bodily damage upon subsequent exposure to that particular antigen.

Hyperthyroidism: A condition resulting from over-function of the thyroid gland.

Hypoallergenic: Refers to products formulated to contain the minimum possible allergens: some people with few allergies can tolerate them well. Severely allergic people can still react to these items.

Hypothyroidism: A condition resulting from under-function of the thyroid gland.

IgA: Immunoglobulin A, an antibody found in secretions associated with mucous membranes.

IgD: Immunoglobulin D, an antibody found on the surface of B-cells.

IgE: Immunoglobulin E, an antibody responsible for immediate hypersensitivity and skin reactions.

IgG: Immunoglobulin G, also known as gammaglobulin, the major antibody in the blood that protects against bacteria and viruses.

IgM: Immunoglobulin M, the first antibody to appear during an immune response.

Immune system: The body's defense system, composed of specialized cells, organs, and body fluids. It has the ability to locate, neutralize, metabolize and eliminate unwanted or foreign substances.

Immunocompromised: A person whose immune system has been damaged or stressed and is not functioning properly.

Immunity: Inherited, acquired, or induced state of being, able to resist a particular antigen by producing antibodies to counteract it. A unique mechanism of the organism to protect and maintain its body against adversity of its surroundings.

Inflammation: The reaction of tissues to injury from trauma, infection, or irritating substances. Affected tissue can be hot, reddened, swollen, and tender.

Inhalant: Any airborne substance small enough to be inhaled into the lungs; eg., pollen, dust, mold, animal danders, perfume, smoke, and smell from chemical compounds.

Intolerance: Inability of an organism to utilize a substance.

Intracellular: Situated within a cell or cells.

Intradermal: method of testing in which a measured amount of antigen is injected between the top layers of the skin.

Ion: An atom that has lost or gained an electron and thus carries an electric charge.

Kinesiology: Science of movement of the muscle.

Latent: Concealed or inactive.

Leukocytes: White blood cells.

Lipids: Fats and oils that are insoluble in water. Oils are liquids in room temperature and fats are solid.

Lymph: A clear, watery, alkaline body fluid found in the lymph vessels and tissue spaces. Contains mostly white blood cells.

Lymphocyte: A type of white blood cell, usually classified as T-or B-cells.

Macrophage: A white blood cell that kills and ingests microorganisms and other body cells.

Masking: Suppression of symptoms due to frequent exposure to a substance to which a person is sensitive.

Mast cells: Large cells containing histamine, found in mucous membranes and skin cells. The histamine in these cells are released during certain allergic reactions.

Mediated: Serving as the vehicle to bring about a phenomenon. For eg., an IgE-mediated reaction is one in which IgE changes cause the symptoms and the reaction to proceed.

Membrane: A thin sheet or layer of pliable tissue that lines a cavity, connects two structures, selective barrier.

Metabolism: Complex chemical and electrical processes in living cells by which energy is produced and life is maintained. New material is assimilated for growth, repair, and replacement of tissues. Waste products are excreted.

Migraine: A condition marked by recurrent severe headaches often on one side of the head, often accompanied by nausea, vomiting, and light aura. These headaches are frequently attributed to food allergy.

Mucous membranes: Moist tissues forming the lining of body cavities that have an external opening, such as the respiratory, digestive, and urinary tracts.

Muscle Response Testing: A testing technique based on kinesiology to test allergies by comparing the strength of a muscle or a group of muscles in the presence and absence of the allergen.

NAET: (Nambudripad's Allergy Elimination Techniques): A technique to eliminate allergies permanently from the body towards the treated allergen. Developed by Dr. Devi S. Nambudripad 1n 1983 and practiced by over 4,500 medical practitioners worldwide. This technique is completely natural, non-invasive, and drug-free. It has been effectively used in treating all types of allergies and problems arising from allergies. It is taught by Dr. Nambudripad in Buena Park, CA. to currently licensed medical practitioners. If you are interested to learn more about NAET, or seminar, please visit the website: www.naet.com.

Nervous system: A network made up of nerve cells, the brain, and the spinal cord, which regulates and coordinates body activities.

Neurotransmitter: A molecule that transmits electrical and/or chemical messages from nerve cell (neuron) to nerve cell or from nerve cell to muscle, secretory, or organ cells.

Nutrients: Vitamins, minerals, amino acids, fatty acids, and sugar (glucose), which are the raw materials needed by the body to provide energy, effect repairs, and maintain functions.

Organic foods: Foods grown in soil free of chemical fertilizers, and without pesticides, fungicides and herbicides.

Overload: The overpowering of the immune system due to massive concurrent exposure or to low level continuous exposure caused by many stresses, including allergens.

Parasite: An organism that depends on another organism (host) for food and shelter, contributing nothing to the survival of the host.

Pathogenic: Capable of causing disease.

Pathology: The scientific study of disease; its cause, processes, structural or functional changes, developments and consequences.

Pathway: The metabolic route used by body systems to facilitate biochemical functions.

Postnasal drip: The leakage of nasal fluids and mucus down into the back of the throat.

Precursor: Anything that proceeds another thing or event, such as physiologically inactive substance that is converted into an active substance that is converted into an active enzyme, vitamin, or hormone.

Prostaglandin: A group of unsaturated, modified fatty acids with regulatory functions.

Radiation: The process of emission, transmission, and absorption of any type of waves or particles of energy, such as light, radio, ultraviolet or X-rays.

Receptor: Special protein structures on cells where hormones, neurotransmitters, and enzymes attach to the cell surface.

Respiratory system: The system that begins with the nostrils and extends through the nose to the back of the throat and into the larynx and lungs.

Rotation diet: A diet in which a particular food and other foods in the same "family" are eaten only once every four to seven days.

Sensitivity: An adaptive state in which a person develops a group of adverse symptoms to the environment, either internal or external. Generally refers to non-IgE reactions.

Serotonin: A constituent of blood platelets and other organs that is released during allergic reactions. It also functions as a neurotransmitter in the body.

Sick building syndrome: (Also known as building materials related illness). This term is used when one or more occupants of a building develops similar symptoms related to some indoor pollutants. Many of these symptoms involve reactions to carpets, formaldehyde, pressed woods, paints, fiber glass, tile work, chemical cleansers, leaking gas from plastic and other synthetic materials.

Steroid: A substance of naturally occurring lipid molecules such as hormones, bile acids, precursors for vitamins, and certain natural drugs, in pharmacology, a synthetic compound used to suppress the action of the immune system.

Stress: Anything that places undue strain upon normal body functions. Stress may be internal in origin (disease, malnutrition, allergic reaction), or external (environmental factors).

Sublingual: Under the tongue, method of testing or treatment in which a measured amount of an antigen or extract is administered under the tongue, behind the teeth. Absorption of the substance is rapid in this way.

Supplement: Nutrient material taken in addition to food in order to satisfy extra demands, effect repair, and prevent degeneration of body systems.

Symptoms: A recognizable change in a person's physical or mental state, that is different from normal function, sensation, or appearance and may indicate a disorder or disease.

Syndrome: A group of symptoms or signs that, occurring together, produce a pattern typical of a particular disorder.

Synthesis: Combining of separate elements and substances to make a new, coherent whole.

Synthetic: Made in a laboratory; not normally produced in nature, or may be a copy of a substance made in nature.

Systemic: Affecting the entire body.

Target organ: The particular organ or system in an individual that will be affected most often by allergic reactions to varying substances.

Tolerance: The capacity of the body to withstand repeated exposure without symptoms.

Toxicity: A poisonous, irritating, or injurious effect resulting when a person ingests or produces a substance in excess of his or her tolerance threshold.

Toxin: Poisonous, irritating, or injurious substance.

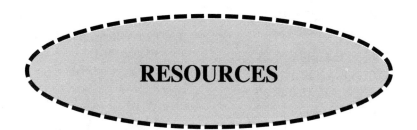

RESOURCES

RESOURCES

Nambudripad Allergy Research Foundation
6714 Beach Blvd
Buena Park, CA 90621
(714)523-0800

NAET Seminars
6714 Beach Blvd
Buena Park, CA 90621
(714)523-8900

Delta Publishing Co.
6714 Beach Blvd.
Buena Park, CA 90621
(714)523-0800

American Environmental Health Foundation
8345 Walnut Hill Circle, Ste. 200
Dallas, TX 75231
(800) 428-2343

For Veterinary NAET

VetNAET.com

Bio Meridian, Inc.
1225 E. Fort Union Blvd., Ste #200
Midvale, UT 84047-1882
(801) 561-4707

Chiro-Tech, Inc
628 Calle Plano
Camarillo, CA 93010
(805) 388-7127

Janice Corporation
198 US Highway 46
Budd Lake, NJ 07828-3001
(800) 526-4237

Non-allergic cotton gloves, bedsheets, and other nonallergic products.

La Chance Release Method
Toby Champion, D.C.
8818 W. Olympic Blvd
Beverly Hills, CA 90211
(310) 273-1221

Neuro Emotional Technique
Dr. Scott Walker
524 2nd Street
Encinitas, CA 02024
(760) 944 1030

Psychoenergetics
Jordan Weiss, M.D.
For seminar and appointments Please call:
Idoheal@aol.com
(949) 263-2362

Autism Outreach project
123 Franklin Corner Road. Ste 215 Lawrenceville, NJ 98648
(609) 895-0190

Autism Research Institute
4182 Adams Ave
San Diego, CA 92116
(619) 281-7165

Autism Society of America
7910 Woodmont Avenue, Ste. 650
Bethesda, MD 200814

National Information Center for Children and Youth with disabilities
PO Box. 1492
Washington, D.C. 20013

Standard Process of Southern California
5611 Palmer way, Ste. F.
Carlsbad, CA 92008
(800) 372-7218
Fax: 800-431-7662
Website: www.spsocal.com
Standard dosages are given below. Dosage for individual child should be determined at the time of administration. Read chapter 9 for proper supplementation. (Call the company for Consultation for further Nutritional Support).

Suggested products:
Allerplex
Antronex
Betaine HCL
Calcium lactate
Cataplex A (Vitamin A)

Cataplex B (B vitamins)
Choline
Congaplex
Drenamin
Immuplex
Inositol
Iplex
Minchex
Mintran
Multizyme
Occulotrophin
Organic Minerals
Ovotrophin
Parotid
Paraplex
Pancreatin
Simplex F
Simplex M
Sesame seed oil
Utrophin
Wheat germ oil

Pure Encapsulation
www.purecaps.com
1-800-753-2277
DL Phenylalanine
Fatty Acids
Antioxidant
Amino Acids

Lotus Herbs
1124 N. Hacienda Blvd
La Puente, CA 91744
(818) 916-1070

These herbal products will be sold to licensed medical practitioners only. Patients should not call the company directly.

Standard dosages are given below. Dosage for individual child should be determined at the time of administration. Read chapter 9 for proper supplementation.

1. Agastahe formula - 1 capsule twice a day with meals
2. Minor bupluerum formula - 1 capsule twice a day
3. Minor blue dragon combination - 1 capsule once or twice a day
4. Siler and platycodon formula - 1 capsule 1 three times a day
5. Minor cinnamon and peony formula - bedwetting, irritability.
6. Hoelen and Schizandra formula - asthma.
7. Tankeui and peony formula - PMS
8. Bupluerum single herb - depression
9. Persica and Rhubarb combination (P.M.S., eczema, acne, hives, warts, dermatitis).

The Herb Finder
P.O.Box 2557
St. George, UT 84771-2557
Phone. (801) 652-9573
Product: Turkey Rhubarb/ Herbal Laxative

BIBLIOGRAPHY

BIBLIOGRAPHY

Ali, Majid M.D. *The Canary and Chronic Fatigue* Life Span Press, New Jersey, 1995

Bender, David, and Bruno Leone *The Environment, Opposing Viewpoints,* Greenhaven Press, San Diego, 1996

Blum, Jeanne Elizabeth *Woman Heal Thyself* Tuttle Co., Inc., Charles E., Boston 1995

Chaitow, Leon. *The Acupuncture Treatment of Pain* Thorsons Publishers Inc., New York 1984

Cousins, Norman. *Head First, The Biology of Hope and the Healing Power of the Human Spirit,* Penguin Books, New York, 1990

East Asian Medical Studies Society. *Fundamentals of Chinese Medicine* Paraadigm Publications, Brookline1985

Fulton, Shaton *The Allergy Self Help Book* Rodale Books, Philadelphia, 1983

Fujihara, Ken, and Hays, Nancy *Common Health Complaints.* Oriental Healing Arts Institute, 1982

Gabriel, Ingrid *Herb Identifier and Handbook* Sterling Publishing Co., Inc., New York 1980

Gach, Michael Reed *Acuppressure's Potent Points* Bantam Books, New York, 1990

Goodheart, George, J *Applied Kinesiology* N.P., 1964

Hsu, Hong-Yen, Ph.D. *Chinese Herb Medicine and Therapy* Oriental Healing Arts Institute, 1982

---. *Commonly Used Chinese Herb Formulas with Illustrations* Oriental Healing Arts Institute, 1982

Heuns, Him-Che *Handbook of Chinese Herbs and Formulae.* Vol V. Los Angeles, 1985

Kirschmann J. D. with L. J. Dunne *Nutrition Almanac* 2nd ed., McGraw Hill Book Co. Copyright 1984

Lyght, Charles E., M.D. and John M. Trapnell, M.D. eds., *The Merck Manual.* 11th ed. Rahway Merck Research Laboratories, 1999

Mc Ilwain, Harris H. M.D., and Debra Fulghum Bruce *The Fibromyalglia Handbook* Holt and Co., New York, 1996

Mindell, Earl. *Vitamin Bible* Warner Books, New York, 1985

Milne, Robert, M.D., Blake More, and Burton Goldberg *An Alternative Medicine Definitive Guide to Headaches* Tiburon, 1997

Nambudripad, Devi S., D.C., L.Ac., Ph.D. *You can reprogram your brain to perfect health* Singer publishing, Palm Springs, CA, 1987

Nambudripad, Devi S., D.C., L.Ac., Ph.D. *Say Good-bye to Illness.* Delta publishing co., Buena Park, CA: 1993, 1999

Nambudripad, Devi S., D.C., L.Ac., Ph.D. *Living Pain Free* - A self-help book using acupressure for pain control. Delta publishing Co., Buena Park, CA, 1997

Nambudripad, Devi S., D.C., L.Ac., Ph.D. *Say Good-bye to ADD and ADHD* Delta publishing Co., Buena Park, CA, 1999

Nambudripad, Devi S., D.C., L.Ac., Ph.D. *The NAET guidebook a companion to Say Good-bye to Illness* . Delta publishing Co., Buena Park, CA: 1993, 94, 95, 96, 97, 98, 99

Nambudripad, Devi S., D.C., L.Ac., Ph.D. *Say Good-bye to Allergy-related Autism* Delta publishing Co., Buena Park, CA, 1999

Northrup, Christiane M.D. *Women's Bodies, Women's Wisdom* Bantam Books, New York, 1998

Pearson, Durk, and Sandy Shaw *The Life Extension Companion* Warner Books, New York, 1984

Kennington & Church. *Food Values of Portions Commonly Used.* J.B. Lippincott Company, 1998

Pert, Candace B., Ph.D. *Molecules of Emotion* New York: Scribner, New York, 1997

Pitchford, Paul *Healing with Whole Foods* North Atlantic Books, Berkeley, 1993

Randolph, Theron, G.,M.D., and Ralph W. Moss, Ph.D. *An Alternative Approach to Allergies* Lippincott and Conwell, New York, 1980

Radetsky, Peter. *Allergic to the Twentieth Century* Boston Little, Brown and Co., Boston, 1997

Rapp, Doris. *Allergy and Your Family* Sterling Publishing Co., New York, 1980.

Rapp, Doris *Is This Your Child?* New York: Quill, William Morrow, 1991

Shanghai College of Traditional Chinese Medicine. *Acupuncture, a Comprehensive Text.*

Shima, Mike. *The Medical I Ching* Blue Poppy Press, Boulder, CO, 1992

Smith, John, H., D.C. *Applied Kinesiology and the Specific Muscle Balancing Technique*

Zong, Linda. *"Chinese Internal Medicine,"* lecture at SAMRA University, Los Angeles, CA. 1985

Case Histories from the Author's private practice,1984-present.

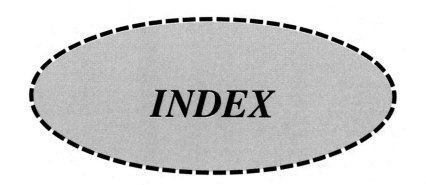

INDEX

Index

ALSO BY DR. NAMBUDRIPAD

The books that tell you all about NAET

Say Good-bye to Allergy-Related Autism
Say Good-bye to ADD and ADHD
Say Good-bye To Illness (English) 2nd ed.
Say Good-bye To Illness (French)
Say Good-bye To Illness (Spanish)
The NAET Guide Book
Living Pain Free

BOOKS ORDER FORM

Name of Book	Price/book	No. of books	Price Total
Say Good-bye to Illness (English)	$24.00	---------------	--------------
Say Good-bye to Illness (French)	$24.00	---------------	--------------
Say Good-bye to Illness (Spanish)	$21.00	---------------	--------------
Say Good-bye ADD & ADHD	$18.00	---------------	--------------
Say Good-bye Allergy Related Autism	$18.00	---------------	--------------
Say Good-bye Children's Allergies	$18.00	---------------	--------------
Living Pain Free	$22.95	--------------	--------------
The NAET Guide Book	$12.00	---------------	--------------

Call 1-(888) 890-0670 or send a check or money order in
the amount of the price plus applicable sales tax and $5.00
shipping and handling to:

    Delta Publishing Company

    6714 Beach Blvd.

    Buena Park, CA 90621

      or, visit our website at:www.naet.com